SI
SOME ▌▌▌▌▌▌▌▌▌▌▌▌▌▌▌▌ *:D*
T0160873

"An exceptional find! There are books about addiction, books about chronic pain, and books about recovery, but it is a rarity to find a book that addresses the three together. *Some Assembly Required* offers the reader a powerful portrayal of the interplay of drug abuse and chronic pain and is equally strong in its emphasis on the tools that offer recovery from both. Dan Mager quickly captures the reader with his gifted use of words, metaphors, and brutal honesty. This is a must-read for anyone, personally or professionally, who wants to understand addiction, living with addiction and chronic pain, and recovery. Educational and thought-provoking—it is an inspiring read."

Claudia Black, PhD
Addiction Specialist
Author of *It Will Never Happen to Me*, *A Hole in the Sidewalk*,
The Truth Begins with You, and coauthor of *Intimate Treason*

"Dan Mager uses his personal and professional experience to illustrate how twelve-step recovery can be combined with mindfulness-based practices, as well as Western psychological theory and psychotherapeutic approaches. Written with insight and humor, this book is a heartfelt story of how the integration of these elements can facilitate the internal shift from chronic avoidance of one's emotional and physical pain to acceptance of it. For those struggling with addiction and chronic pain, and the professionals who desire to help them, *Some Assembly Required* is an important read."

John C. Friel, PhD
MN and NV Licensed Psychologist
Author of *The Power and Grace Between Nasty or Nice: Replacing Entitlement, Narcissism, and Incivility with Knowledge, Caring, and Genuine Self-Esteem* and *The 7 Best Things Happy Couples Do*

"Anyone searching for an interesting education in the chronic pain and addiction genres will find *Some Assembly Required* a must-read. I especially appreciate Dan Mager's unique perspective and broad-based approach to recovery and living with both addiction and chronic pain in a way that works for him, rather than against him. Starting with the Introduction, I was immediately brought into his turbulent journey and fall from grace, and then how he marched through fear to find hope and healing. Dan's way of illustrating the progression and accompanying internal dialogues of active addiction is incredibly powerful. What a great book!"

Jason Z W Powers, MD
Chief Medical Officer
Right Step, Spirit Lodge, and San Cristobal of Elements Behavioral Health
Author of *When the Servant Becomes the Master*

"Dan Mager has written an instructive tale about his struggle with addiction and chronic pain and the power of denial, while offering hope and guidance in sharing his path to recovery."

David E. Smith, MD
Founder of Haight-Ashbury Free Medical Clinics of San Francisco
Past President of American Society of Addiction Medicine
Chief of Addiction Medicine, Newport Academy
Author of *Unchain Your Brain*

[SOME ASSEMBLY REQUIRED]

[SOME ASSEMBLY REQUIRED]

A Balanced Approach to Recovery
from Addiction and Chronic Pain

DAN MAGER

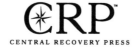

CENTRAL RECOVERY PRESS

Central Recovery Press (CRP) is committed to publishing exceptional materials addressing addiction treatment, recovery, and behavioral healthcare topics, including original and quality books, audio/visual communications, and web-based new media. Through a diverse selection of titles, we seek to contribute a broad range of unique resources for professionals, recovering individuals and their families, and the general public.

For more information, visit **www.centralrecoverypress.com.**

Publisher: Central Recovery Press
3321 N. Buffalo Drive
Las Vegas, NV 89129

18 17 16 15 14 13   1 2 3 4 5

ISBN: 978-1-937612-25-2 (paper)
978-1-937612-26-9 (e-book)

Author photo by Beth Kovac. Used with permission.

Grateful Dead lyrics by Robert Hunter and John Barlow; © copyright Ice Nine Publishing Company. Used with permission.

Quotations from *The Places That Scare You: A Guide to Fearlessness in Difficult Times,* Pema Chödrön, 2001 and *The Wisdom of No Escape and the Path of Loving-Kindness,* Pema Chödrön, 1991. Reprinted by arrangement with Shambhala Publications, Inc., Boston, MA. www.shambhala.com.

Publisher's Note: This is a memoir; a work based on facts recorded to the best of the author's memory. Our books represent the experiences and opinions of our authors only. Every effort has been made to ensure that events, institutions, and statistics presented in our books as facts are accurate and up-to-date. To protect their privacy, the names of some of the people and institutions in this book have been changed.

This book also contains general information about chronic pain, addiction, and addiction treatment. The information is not medical advice, and should not be treated as such. CRP makes no representations or warranties in relation to the medical information in this book; this book is not an alternative to medical advice from your doctor or other professional healthcare provider. If you have any specific questions about any medical matter you should consult your doctor or other professional healthcare provider. You should never delay seeking medical advice, disregard medical advice, or discontinue medical treatment because of information in this or any book.

Cover and interior design and layout by Sara Streifel, Think Creative Design

To my daughters, who have taught me a depth of love
I never knew existed, and who continue to teach me
what unconditional love really means.

To my parents, who only wanted the best for me,
and have always loved me to the best of their ability.

[TABLE OF CONTENTS]

Foreword by Mel Pohl, MD, FASAM ... ix

Acknowledgments ... xv

Introduction ... xvii

Chapter One   **In Through the Out Door** ... 1

Chapter Two   **Start Me Up** ... 9

Chapter Three   **Through the Looking Glass** ... 27

Chapter Four   **If You Meet the Buddha, say Hello** ... 39

Chapter Five   **A Personal Prison in Private Purgatory** ... 51

Chapter Six   **No Matter Where You Go, There You Are** ... 67

Chapter Seven   **You Can't Save Your Face and Your Ass at the Same Time** ... 73

Chapter Eight   **Crisis Creates Opportunity** ... 89

Chapter Nine   **Vegas, Baby** ... 103

Chapter Ten   **One Foot in Front of the Other** ... 121

Chapter Eleven   **An Imperfectly Perfect Support System** ... 131

Chapter Twelve   **Would You Rather Be Right or Would You Rather Be Happy?** ... 147

Chapter Thirteen   **From Awareness to Action**   161

Chapter Fourteen   **Being Here Now**   175

Chapter Fifteen   **Pain Is Inevitable; Suffering Is Optional**   189

Chapter Sixteen   **Personality Challenges and Spiritual Principles**   211

Chapter Seventeen   **Roots then Wings**   229

Chapter Eighteen   **Spiritual Awakenings Come in Many Different Colors**   241

Chapter Nineteen   **There Is No Graduation**   253

Endnotes   265

References   269

[FOREWORD]

By themselves, addiction and chronic pain can be debilitating. When brought together, they comprise extremely complicated co-occurring disorders. In *Some Assembly Required: A Balanced Approach to Recovery from Addiction and Chronic Pain,* Dan Mager has written an extraordinary book that addresses both of these conditions. As a result of my work at Las Vegas Recovery Center (LVRC) I have seen the many sides that Dan artfully describes in his journey from addiction to recovery, from a life of chronic pain to pain recovery.

Addiction is among the most serious public health problems in the United States. In 2010, an estimated 22.1 million persons aged twelve or older were classified with substance dependence or abuse in the past year—8.7 percent of the population aged twelve or older.[1]

In 2009, drug overdose exceeded motor vehicle accidents as a cause of death, killing at least 37,485 people nationwide, according to data from the US Centers for Disease Control and Prevention. Propelled by dramatic increases in prescription pain medication overdoses, this represents the first time that drugs have accounted for more fatalities than traffic accidents since the government started tracking drug-induced deaths in 1979. Overdoses of prescription opioids now cause more deaths than heroin and cocaine combined.[2]

Pain affects more Americans than diabetes, heart disease, and cancer *combined.*[3] And 25 percent of the US population is affected by chronic pain, according to estimates from the National Center for Health Statistics.[4] The annual cost of chronic pain in the United States, including healthcare expenses, lost income, and lost productivity, is estimated to be $100 billion.[5] By far, the most prevalent treatment for both acute and chronic pain is narcotic medications, primarily opioids, such as oxycodone (Percocet, Oxycontin), hydrocodone (Vicodin, Lortab), morphine (MScontin), methadone, and fentanyl (Duragesic, Actiq). The quantity of prescription pain medications sold to pharmacies, hospitals, and doctors' offices was four times larger in 2010 than in 1999. Enough opioids were prescribed in 2010 to medicate every American adult around-the-clock for one month.[6]

There is no data to confirm that using opioids beyond three months for chronic noncancer pain is an efficacious treatment. The rational way to prescribe opioids for chronic pain is as a trial with closely monitored results. As doctors, we need to give enough medication to decrease pain, when possible, but we must remain mindful that for some, stimulating the brain's reward center will lead to problems including addiction. And we ought to use good clinical judgment by taking people off of opioids if their function is not improving. There are many potential problems with opioids. Their side effects include cognitive diminution, constipation, and opioid-induced hyperalgesia, to name just a few. Over time tolerance and physical dependence develop, and of course, the feelings of euphoria that opioid use can evoke in some make these medications potentially addictive.

Prescription drug abuse is by far the fastest-growing drug problem in the United States, and abuse of and addiction to the opioid medications prescribed for pain (the so-called painkillers) are at the forefront of this trend. More than 12 million people reported using prescription opioids nonmedically in 2010—in other words, using them without a prescription and/or specifically for the feelings of euphoria they cause.[7] The misuse and abuse of these drugs was responsible for more than 475,000 emergency department visits in 2009, a number that nearly doubled in just five years.[8]

In 2011, in response to this epidemic of prescription drug abuse, the White House Office of National Drug Control Policy (ONDCP) released an action plan that combines public health and public safety components, including new federal requirements aimed at educating the medical community about proper prescribing practices. At the invitation of ONDCP, I had the privilege of serving as a consultant for this prescription drug abuse initiative.

Addiction is a disease of the brain's reward system and is mediated by dopamine and other neurotransmitters. Addiction drives the need to take substances in pursuit of neurochemical reward. Chronic pain syndrome is a phenomenon described by the International Pain Society as pain that won't go away—a persistent irritation that can't be turned off and may become quite debilitating. The symptoms of addiction include compulsive substance use, depression and anxiety, sleep disturbance, physical problems, significant stress, and functional disability. Chronic pain often has the same set of symptoms, minus the compulsive substance use.

However, if you have both conditions, each one feeds on the other, so that functional disability with pain is made worse by addiction, and sleep disturbance is made worse because of withdrawal, and depression and anxiety are exacerbated by pain, and people use more drugs in the attempt to medicate their physical and emotional pain. When addiction and chronic pain co-occur, these conditions essentially activate each other continuously. There is continued use despite increasing harm, combined with craving. Craving for people with chronic pain and addiction is based around having pain. That's what draws them to continue to use. Opioids relieve both physical and emotional pain for the moment, but eventually backfire, as *Some Assembly Required* depicts with painstaking clarity.

I commonly hear from my patients with chronic pain that "I can only be okay if I take something to relieve my pain," even when the benefit has become minimal and transient, and with time the effects only diminish further. Like many with chronic pain, Dan truly believed that he couldn't live without opioids.

With chronic pain comes the experience of suffering, and suffering is often more influential than the pain itself. Twenty-five hundred years ago, the Buddha said: "When touched with a feeling of pain, the ordinary uninstructed person sorrows, grieves, laments, beats his breast, and becomes distraught. So he feels two pains, physical and mental. Just as if they were to shoot a man with an arrow and, right afterward, were to shoot him with another one, so that he would feel the pains of two arrows." The second arrow is suffering, and that is the overwhelming experience of chronic pain, which is well-characterized in this book.

Fueled by a sense of uniqueness and of being different, helping professionals are often the last to get treatment. With irony and dramatic accuracy, Dan details his parallel journey as a behavioral health/addiction treatment professional and addicted person with all the attendant denial, rationalization, dishonesty, and ambivalence. In describing his process of transcending a professional know-it-all attitude in surrendering to the truth and taking the difficult and necessary steps toward recovery and self-discovery, Dan evidences an honest, self-aware, and realistic view of himself.

Some Assembly Required blends a wonderful matrix of clinical and personal observations about the process of addiction and recovery. It discusses the commonalities between Western psychological theories, certain psychotherapeutic approaches, twelve-step recovery, and Taoism and Buddhism, and provides a comprehensive review of psychological and physical interventions for chronic pain. Dan articulates the complex interplay of thoughts (in the forms of negative self-talk, catastrophization, resistance, and self-judgment) and feelings (such as shame, guilt, anger, fear, depression, and anxiety) associated with his conditions, consistent with what I have observed in many patients who suffer from co-occurring pain and addiction.

As *Some Assembly Required* conveys, there are cognitive-behavioral and mindfulness-based ways to reduce both physical and emotional pain. Basically, if you think differently about your pain and/or you act differently in response to your pain, you have less pain. This is an important component of our pain recovery model at the Las Vegas Recovery Center and Central Recovery Treatment. Pain recovery is about balance. It involves the way we think, how we cope with feelings, how our body is functioning, and our spirituality. The net result is that people have relationships that are enhanced and much greater involvement in positive actions and behaviors. Nonmedication treatments are really all about movement: exercise, release of tissue adhesions through massage, yoga, chi kung, Reiki's nontouch, energy work, and acupuncture.

What we see consistently in our program is that people give up opioids, and they go from a state of depression, despondency, and disability to a state of freedom they didn't think was possible. It is possible to recover from the co-occurring conditions of chronic pain and addiction and live a better life. It can be very tough to get there, but it's the closest thing to miracle work I've ever seen in my thirty-two years of clinical practice.

Some Assembly Required will be of benefit to anyone who struggles with addiction and chronic pain, as well as the professionals who treat them. It is a story of hope and success in the face of disabling illnesses: addiction and chronic pain.

Mel Pohl, MD, FASAM
Vice President of Medical Affairs
Medical Director
Las Vegas Recovery Center

[ACKNOWLEDGMENTS]

There are many people who have directly and indirectly contributed to this project and my heartfelt appreciation extends to all of them. The task of formalizing this list of acknowledgments is inherently intimidating by virtue of the inevitability of certain omissions. There are many thanks to give.

To Nancy Schenck, Executive Editor of CRP and editor for this project, whose guidance and friendship is a great gift. Clearly, one of the reasons I was brought to Las Vegas was for her to be part of my life and my recovery.

To my other talented CRP teammates: Valerie Killeen, Managing Editor, and my walking partner at work, as well as a walking example of professionalism and humility; Helen O'Reilly, Senior Editor and human dictionary; Daniel Kaelin, Editorial Coordinator and permissions guru; Eliza Tutellier, Assistant Editor, who did a wonderful backup edit for this book; and Patrick Hughes, Sales and Marketing Manager, ace book pimp, and cinematic savant.

To Bob Gray, CRP Publisher, whose efforts facilitate our mission.

To Stuart Smith, whose vision and support make this book and all the important work we do at Central Recovery Press possible.

To Mel Pohl, MD, FASAM, for composing the Foreword to this book. To be able to collaborate on projects such as this with the renowned physician who met me at my nadir is a stirring example of what is possible in recovery.

To Claudia Black, PhD, whose groundbreaking work on dysfunctional family systems I utilized with clients as an addiction treatment professional, for her kind feedback and generous support of this project.

To my most excellent colleagues at Central Recovery and Central Recovery Treatment, especially: Debbie Champine, Joni Baumgart, Doyne Pickett, Bill Peiffer, Paul Hinshaw, Travis Shephard, Tony Carter, Dave Lawrence, Greg Pergament, and Alvin Elliot.

To my informal reviewers, Margie Williams, MA, LPC, dear friend and colleague, whose path and mine have had so much in common; and Beth Kovac, my beautiful (inside and out) partner.

To my mentors in behavioral health, most notably: Wendy Yalowitz, MSW, LCSW, my first post-master's supervisor from whom I learned so much about the art of psychotherapy; Dave Glaser, MSW, LCSW, my East Coast Grateful Dead concert-going buddy, who taught me the ropes of clinical supervision and administration; and Susan Rubin, PhD, MSW, who showed me what courageous leadership in the face of political pressure looks like, and was instrumental in helping me refine my management skills. Their guidance and support have been an enduring resource.

To Frank Szabo, for the many extensive discussions we had that clarified and enriched my understanding of recovery.

To Phil F, who loved me when I had little capacity to love myself, and foresaw this book long before I ever did.

To Jimmy S, a living example of how to walk a spiritual path, even on burning coals in bare feet.

To Alan Trist at Ice Nine Publishing Company, who immediately and generously granted my request to use Grateful Dead lyrics in chapter epigraphs for this book. I am honored to be able to quote from songs that have meant so much to me and have been so close to my heart for so long.

[INTRODUCTION]

There is no shortage of autobiographical stories that describe the horrors of addiction. Many of these also depict people's journeys into recovery. Some of these narrative self-portraits have been painted by those who rose from the ashes of their active addiction to find recovery and go on to become addiction counselors. The usual sequence of events is active addiction to recovery to counselor/therapist/helping professional. This story is a little different. Like no small number of things in my life, I got it ass-backward insofar as I was a behavioral health professional, working in high-level management capacities for many years, plenty of which were in addiction treatment settings—*before* I entered recovery.

As I moved up the promotional ladder, I transitioned from full-time direct practice as a therapist to providing clinical supervision and teaching treatment approaches and techniques to dozens of counselors, therapists, interns, and other staff. I was responsible for overseeing the clinical operations of (in succession) a residential addiction treatment center for adolescents, a hospital-based inpatient addiction treatment program for adults, and multi-program outpatient treatment services for adults, children, and families—all while I was in active addiction. In these settings, I was highly regarded as a practitioner and administrator.

Of all the twists and turns my life has taken, I never expected to be confronted by the challenges and complexities that lie at the nexus of addiction and chronic pain. As an experienced clinician with a master's degree in social work and advanced training and credentialing in clinical hypnosis, I knew a thing or two about the connection between thoughts, emotions, and physical pain.

I had treated others' suffering from chronic pain with unanticipated success using hypnosis. However, with the onset of my own chronic pain condition and its intersection with the addiction that had long predated it, all my professional knowledge and experience faded away. For all rational and practical purposes, it was nonexistent to me.

I allowed myself to become utterly dependent upon the prevailing conventional Western medical approach to pain management with its merry-go-round of opioid painkillers, lumbar epidural steroid injections, occasional episodes of physical therapy, and the ever-looming option of spinal fusion. I effectively assumed the position of victim. And in doing so, I submissively succumbed to the admonitions of my doctors (all extremely experienced, skilled, and well-intentioned) and relinquished sports and other physical activities that potentially put me at risk for further injury. As a lifelong athlete, this was an especially devastating loss. As I became more sedentary, my physical functioning only deteriorated further, and the vicious circle of chronic pain and addiction to the narcotic medications prescribed for it progressively hijacked my priorities, and my world became smaller and smaller.

In fact, my need for the opioid painkillers reawakened an addiction to narcotics that had been in hibernation for over fifteen years. I convinced myself that I had somehow outgrown the use of such "hard" drugs while I settled into a long-term pattern of marijuana and alcohol maintenance. My chronic pain gave me medical sanction to dive into my real dope of choice, as the serpent of my addiction awoke full force and began to devour me.

Physical pain became my main river of feeling. All other emotions—sadness, fear, anxiety, hurt, guilt, frustration, anger, depression, etc.—were tributaries that ran into it, fed it, and increased its flow and power. These uncomfortable, often painful emotions became harder to distinguish from one another, and my inability to tolerate them created a truckload of internal stress that only made my pain worse—inviting, no, demanding, that I use more and more opioids.

The disease of addiction is known for being "cunning, baffling, and powerful." It is also exquisitely patient, as well as treacherous and seductive in the ways it attempts to convince those who suffer from it that they don't have it. Ironically, as long as my addiction was active, my education and professional experience obstructed my ability to see it for what it was, to admit to it, and in turn, to take responsibility for it and seek help.

My internal self-talk kept feeding me various reassuring lines of bullshit about how different I was from other addicts, especially those who I had worked with in my professional capacities. I was definitely *not* like "them." After all, I was on the other side of the desk. And with the injection of chronic pain into the landscape of my addiction, I easily relied on the rationalization that my using was medically necessary. My head was relentless in arguing that I was *not* an addict, in spite of knowing that addiction is an equal opportunity illness that can afflict anyone, regardless of race, community, socioeconomic status, or occupation.

It wasn't until I got to a dark and desperate enough place, where I could no longer avoid a reality that had long been evident, went into treatment myself, and began to work a program of recovery that my professional background began to shift from impediment to asset. Once I started to actually do something about my addiction and make some significant changes in the way I was living, I realized that my recovery could benefit from my knowledge and skills.

My professional experience had the potential to be a strength in that it gave me a well-developed frame of reference for the therapeutic process of change. By therapeutic, I mean in the most general reparative, restorative sense. I had a solid understanding of the processes of learning, growing, and healing—which happen to be intimately related to recovery from both addiction and chronic pain. Admittedly, this frame of reference and understanding was primarily intellectual, but nonetheless it was a valuable resource to build upon.

My behavioral health background also had great potential to be an ongoing obstacle. In spite of the wreckage my active addiction left in its wake, my thinking could have cajoled me into continuing to believe that I was still somehow unique and so much less messed up than my peers in treatment. My head might have convinced me that I could use my professional bona fides to fall back on what I already knew, or to believe that I knew it all, or at least to believe that I knew "enough." My internal voice could have talked me into acting as if I didn't have to put in the inherently difficult and extremely challenging daily work of recovery—that it really wasn't necessary for me to practice the open-mindedness, willingness, and humility (among many, many other ingredients) required to look at and do things differently.

Wrapping my mind around the need to give up my primary coping mechanism of over thirty years, in addition to finding alternative ways to live with a chronic pain condition, has been a profoundly uncomfortable and often arduous process. However, this is a beautiful, warm, sunny day on a tropical beach compared to the *hellacious* challenge of truly accepting it at the much deeper level of my heart. Only by embracing the process of recovery (or any process of meaningful change for that matter) with my heart can I apply its principles in the moment-to-moment unfolding of my life.

Because addiction and chronic pain have physical, mental, emotional, and spiritual elements, recovery from both requires mental, emotional, physical, and spiritual components. Successful, sustained recovery requires balance between these four life domains, as well as within each of them.

Recovery has gifted me with opportunities to see beyond the limitations of the lenses of my past experiences:

- to recognize how aspects of bio-psycho-social development and specific theories of psychology connect with the twelve-step approach and can enrich my understanding of the recovery process; and

- to appreciate how certain counseling models and approaches can dovetail with twelve-step philosophy and programs, along with particular spiritual perspectives and mindfulness practices, to create the synergy of a whole that is greater, more powerful, and more therapeutic than the sum of its parts.

Putting these pieces together to change how I relate to myself, to others, and to the world is an extraordinary undertaking, requiring no small amount of mental, emotional, and spiritual renovation. Keeping my heart fully engaged as I learn how to be okay with myself, as well as with life on its own terms, in this moment, in order to continue my growth and healing, one day at a time, is a Herculean task. And, there is no adventure more worthwhile.

This book is part memoir, part self-help guide, and part clinical-psychoeducational exposition on addiction and chronic pain. As you will notice, the material alternates between these three elements, shifting gears as it moves from the personal to the professional and back again. It provides a framework for recovery from these life-altering co-occurring disorders that has served me well, and which I hope will be of value to others.

I have had the benefit of living in different areas of the United States. I've made cross-country trips of 2,000–3,000 miles many times. I've driven the 3,000 miles from Long Island to San Francisco (driving our van off the side of Interstate 80 and nearly down an embankment in western Pennsylvania in a pot-induced daze in 1980), and flown from Phoenix to Tel Aviv (fortified by two liters of wine and a pocket full of pills). Yet, the longest distance I have ever traveled is that from my head to my heart.

chapter one

[IN THROUGH THE OUT DOOR]

"The blessing lies close to the wound."

AFRICAN PROVERB

It was the third day of my medically managed detoxification when Allison, one of the counselors, came over and sat down next to me in the treatment center dining room. Speaking softly she said, "I don't know if you remember me, but when you were Vice President of Counseling at Jewish Family & Children's Service in Tucson, you accepted me for an MSW (Masters in Social Work) field placement."

Taken aback, I struggled to bring my vision into sharper focus. I was a mess—negotiating the dense fog of a complex combination of medications while treading water in a stormy sea of self-recrimination and self-loathing. Massive waves of shame, embarrassment, remorse, and guilt buffeted me, knocking me around, turning me upside down and inside out. Although I had seen her around the facility and had even attended a group she facilitated, no bells of familiarity rang . . . until then. Looking at her intently, I suddenly recognized her. "Yes, of course I remember you."

As the once-upon-a-time Vice President of Counseling, I had final approval on all field placements in the Counseling Services Department, and occasionally interviewed applicants directly. A little over three years prior to this "reunion," I had interviewed Allison. She was a second year MSW student from the Arizona State University satellite program in Tucson who impressed me as possessing the intelligence, maturity, and personality prerequisites that are so important in a fast-paced, team-oriented behavioral health services environment. I had specifically recommended that Barbara, one of our two clinical supervisors, be assigned as her field instructor.

Allison spoke to me with kindness and compassion, never asking nor even implying, "What the hell happened to you?" while the voice inside my head revved up, not so much in distress, as in deep sadness and resignation: "Holy shit. I really can't fucking believe just how far I've fallen." If I didn't already have enough evidence of how the consequences of my three decades of active addiction had finally caught up with me and kicked my ass every which way, here was another compelling brick in that wall.

In what I interpreted as an attempt to be respectful and sensitive to my dizzying descent from grace, Allison told me that she would not disclose to other staff, including my assigned counselor, that she knew me from such a different time and place. I thanked her for this extraordinary (and not altogether appropriate) consideration and let her know that the staff needed to know, and that I would tell my counselor about our shared history, as well as my fellow clients. At age forty-seven, I had at last reached the point where I could no longer continue to live a double life. It had been a long time coming.

The walls of active addiction had been closing in on me, gradually and progressively, for what seemed like forever. During the last few years, the more energy I invested in keeping those walls at bay, the more I lived in fear of being found out. Not only was I doing everything possible to keep others from discovering this truth, I was also going to great lengths to keep it at a safe distance from myself. This was an exhausting and grim cycle wherein the harder I labored to protect myself from the conscious awareness of what I had become, the more intrusive and unavoidable that awareness became. Eventually, all of my stratagems—external and internal—failed.

Throughout my life I had taken many serious risks, and there were times when the perpetual pursuit of the ways and means to procure and use drugs had placed me squarely in the path of great potential physical, legal, and in later years, professional harm. And yet, the very thought of admitting that I was an "addict" scared the shit out of me. There was abject dread intrinsic to admitting it to myself, much less to anyone else. This fear fueled, at times, a desperate need to defend myself psychologically against an increasingly inescapable reality.

Among the most challenging and painful experiences I've had was to find myself in a group setting in treatment as a patient in early November of 2006, and say aloud for the first time, "I'm Dan, and I'm an addict." I felt so raw; it was as if my skin had been peeled off. I don't ever remember feeling so completely exposed, so excruciatingly vulnerable (at least not as an adult). My voice shook and I don't know if my body literally trembled, but it sure as hell felt like it did. I had consciously and unconsciously avoided that admission for decades—denying, minimizing, rationalizing, and intellectualizing to keep the reality of my addiction hidden behind a wall of steadfast self-protection.

My wife had long known what I was incapable of acknowledging. To her exasperation and enduring credit, she had tried intermittently since the early 1980s, even before we were married, to get me to seek help.

"You're a drug addict, and you need to do something about it."

"I'm not a drug addict. I recently graduated from college with honors and a double major." (Never mind that I never quite completed the second major because the required senior thesis went unfinished, and my addiction was instrumental in keeping it that way.)

"You're a drug addict, and you need to do something about it."

"I can't be a drug addict. I've been accepted to every master's program I applied to, including Columbia University and NYU."

"You're a drug addict, and you need to do something about it."

"I'm definitely not a drug addict. I just completed one of the most prestigious MSW programs in the country."

"You're a drug addict, and you need to do something about it."

"There's no way I'm a drug addict. I was just promoted to clinical director of a substance abuse treatment program."

"You're a drug addict, and you need to do something about it."

"I'm not a drug addict. I'm an adjunct professor teaching undergraduate college courses on psychology and substance abuse."

"You're a drug addict, and you need to do something about it."

"I'm not a drug addict. I help drug addicts."

And that only takes me to 1997. I still had nine years of active addiction ahead, and my chronic pain condition had yet to make its appearance and further distort my sense of proportion. Deep down, in the remote recesses of my consciousness, a part of me had always known that she was right. But as much as I could, I kept this awareness buried in a box on the top shelf all the way in the back of my mind's closet. Although occasionally this awareness would escape from its container to haunt me, it rarely saw the light of day. I wasn't ready to do anything differently

. . . until I was. Things had to get bad; and then they had to get worse—much worse—before I got to the point where I could no longer continue as I had been.

Prior to the culmination of my devolution from treatment provider to treatment patient, my active addiction went through many phases. Some were higher risk, more intense, and sped up the disease's progression; others were less overtly hazardous and precipitated a slower pace of progression. I had been in one of those latter "safer" phases for about fifteen years when the onset of a chronic pain condition set me on a slippery slope that turbo-charged my acceleration toward self-demolition.

In the years prior to the onset of my chronic pain, the state of my addiction was analogous to riding a Flexible Flyer sled down a gently sloping snow-covered hill (as I did during winters as a kid growing up on Long Island, NY). There was always the slight possibility of running into a tree or the sled overturning, but the chances of serious injury were minimal. By contrast, the medically prescribed treatment for my chronic pain put me in the front seat of a bobsled speeding over an icy track.

My experience during the more perilous phases of my addiction was like that of an Olympic bobsled driver—intimately acquainted with whipping around sharp turns at dangerously high speeds while fighting to control the vehicle and maintain its balance in order to keep it from flipping over or going off the track and crashing. It's an exhilarating and often anxiety-inducing rush unto itself, separate from, though related to the neurochemical detonation of mind-and mood-altering drugs in the brain. Each time on the track risks potential disaster, and the more runs even elite-level bobsledders attempt, the more likely it is that they will, at some point, crash.

Such crashes can be devastating, often resulting in serious injury or death. No matter how experienced and skilled we are (or believe ourselves to be), no matter how well we have our shit together (or think we do), the odds have a way of eventually catching up with us.

I found resourcefully manipulative and creatively dishonest ways of keeping that bobsled on the track past the point where it was beyond my capacity to control it. The grossly disparate parts of my life that I had worked so hard to keep isolated from one another—successful behavioral health professional, committed, loving, responsible husband and parent, and dissembling, practicing addict—increasingly began to collide. Ultimately, the walls that separated them crumbled and fell, leaving my sense of self, my family, and my career buried in an avalanche of rubble.

As the shitstorm blew up, it splattered me with the consequences of my choices and actions and my defenses started to fall apart. The psychological bulwarks that had protected me from too much conscious contact with the reality of my addiction and allowed it to continue came undone. The awareness that I was an addict could no longer be suppressed. It refused to stay put in the designated compartments of my cognitive closet and was now in my face, unleashing a torrent of mental, emotional, and spiritual anguish and demanding acknowledgment.

Nearly twenty years of post-master's experience in counseling, many of which were in addiction treatment settings, was a double-edged sword. Being familiar with the formal criteria for "substance dependence"—drug addiction, in the parlance of the fourth edition of the bible of diagnosis, the Diagnostic and Statistical Manual of Mental Disorders (DSM) (the fifth edition, due for release in May of 2013, will include a diagnostic category for "addiction")—intellectually, I knew that I qualified. At the same time, my expertise continued to seduce me into believing that I was different because I was a "professional," who, until the bitter end of my using, as impaired as I often was, still received stellar performance evaluations and demonstrated an ability to be effective with both staff and clients.

Change rarely comes easily. Making significant change in any aspect of life is really hard, as well as frightening. The greater the change, the higher the degree of difficulty and fear associated with it. Similar to physical workouts, there is a general correlation between the discomfort we are willing to go through and the outcomes we get—"no pain, no gain." The greatest growth comes from pushing ourselves to go beyond the boundaries of the boxes of familiarity and comfort that we have constructed.

A lot of people stay in situations that are painful and unhealthy because they are familiar with the pain of their specific situation. They are well acquainted with it and know exactly how it works and what the results will be. Their current circumstances provide an incongruous comfort based on familiarity, predictability, and certainty. Even if it is horrible, they know what to expect. Usually, this dynamic operates under the surface of conscious awareness such that, even when someone knows that change is necessary and wants to change, he or she seems unable to do so.

What we know is always much more comfortable than what we don't know, despite the potential other options may have to be better and healthier. The attraction and power of familiarity and the comfort it provides is not to be underestimated. This is the essence of the emotional cement that keeps people stuck in circumstances that are unsatisfying, unhealthy, and sometimes even dangerous, such as living situations; jobs/career paths; relationships, including those that are abusive or violent; and active addiction.

The fear of the unknown and the uncertainty that goes hand-in-hand with it is natural, normal, and understandable. Sometimes, it can be debilitating. For many people—in this case, me—change occurs only when the pain of staying the same outweighs the fear of doing something different.

After using for over thirty-five years, and using one or more substances virtually every day for thirty years, I could no longer live with drugs. But, I couldn't see how I could possibly live without them. I was terrified by the prospect of trying to negotiate life's emotional and physical minefields without mind- and/or mood-altering chemicals. I felt like I was being dropped into a foreign and uncharted wilderness in the middle of the night, during a snowstorm, without GPS, a compass, or even a map. I had no idea how to navigate this completely unfamiliar territory. I just knew that I couldn't do it alone.

chapter two

[START ME UP]

*"Holding on to anger is like grasping a hot coal
with the intent of throwing it at someone else;
you are the one who gets burned."*

THE BUDDHA

Past experiences, especially those from childhood, are legacies that can leave lasting imprints upon us. The messages we receive growing up in our family of origin, neighborhood, and community cast long shadows over how we learned to relate to ourselves, to others, and to the world. As a result, my fundamental patterns of thinking, expressing emotion, decision-making, and behaving were established long before the onset of my active addiction.

The images are seared into my memory with crystal clarity, though everything floats in shades of gray. Even beyond the black-and-white television broadcast, the entire tableau was monochromatic like the all too common metropolitan New York day where the overcast is so thick you can feel the gloominess and the weight of the air on your skin. Although I was focused on the screen, I was also intently watching my mother watching and reacting in real time as the horse-drawn caisson bearing the body of the thirty-fifth president of the United States made its excruciatingly slow march as the centerpiece of the funeral procession.

The clip-clop of the horses' hooves on the street surface seemed to echo off the walls of our living room. Although I could figure out from the overall aesthetic that this was a somber occasion, through observing my mother I began to sense how immense and tragic an event this was. Her sobbing filled the entire house, filling my small world. I hesitantly asked questions in an attempt to better understand what I was witnessing on TV and in the room, but even though she was there, she really wasn't. Under her crying, she just kept repeating to no one in particular, "He was such a great man," over and over like some sort of mantra. Indeed, as I would come to learn, John F. Kennedy (for all of the flaws and self-indulgences that would be revealed many years later) was a figure of remarkable promise and possibility.

My mother's sadness engulfed me as my attention shifted back and forth between the pictures on the TV screen and her responses to them. I don't know how long the television coverage of the funeral lasted, but it seemed to go on for days. Everything else faded away and I became so present-centered that I entered a state of trance, a state that would later become very familiar to me. If I listen closely, I can still hear the sound of horse hooves on concrete.

The assassination of JFK was a national trauma that became fused into the emotional DNA of America. His death would come to represent, not only a loss of national innocence, but also the death of a collective sense of unlimited potential. Of course I had no real sense of any of this at the time, but somehow, at least as far as the weight of the moment, I got it. Another aspect of my experience of that dreary yet mesmerizing day that would become familiar to me was that, emotionally, I was on my own.

It was late November 1963, and I was four-and-a-half years old. By this time, my younger brother was nearly three, and the older of my two younger sisters was almost eight months old. My youngest sister would be born four months later, just 360 days separating the two of them. Doing the math reveals that I am the oldest of four children born to my parents in less than six years. As my father would delight in saying to anyone who expressed interest in this peculiar form of family planning, "We held at two pair and yielded to a full house!"

My parents didn't believe in wasting time. When they announced to their own families that they were getting married all of six weeks after they first met, my maternal grandmother asked the obvious question, "Do they have to?" As the family narrative has it, they weren't pregnant, it was simply a love-at-first-sight whirlwind courtship that enveloped them in its inevitability: they knew. My parents have always insisted that all of their children were fully planned. Every family has its mythology.

The very first indication that I had a potential predisposition to using drugs came when I was two years old. When my father returned home from work each evening, his ritual included a glass of Scotch. As the story goes, according to both my parents, even at this tender age, I displayed an obvious attraction to the alcohol—reaching for his Scotch and wanting to taste it myself.

This occurred on a nightly basis for some time and became increasingly annoying. My father was impressed by my persistence, and ultimately determined that one taste would be aversive enough to cure me of my interest. So, with my mother's reluctant consent, he allowed me a sip. To their complete astonishment, as they both report it (it has always been a rare occurrence—kind of like a solar eclipse—when the two of them remember the same incident exactly the same way), my verbatim response was as follows: "Hot . . . burn . . . good . . . more!" That might have been a clue.

My father was a workaholic who regularly got home long after the rest of the family had eaten dinner. As a manufacturer's representative in the furniture industry, he worked on commission and was effectively self-employed. His work days were spent driving throughout the New York-New Jersey-Connecticut metropolitan area to see customers, and when he wasn't on the road, he was often in his office at our home in Oyster Bay on the north shore of Nassau County about thirty miles east of Manhattan. Even in the mid-1960s, we had two phone lines; one was the regular home phone and the other was for my father's business. When the business phone rang, answering it became the highest priority; everything else took a backseat until whatever business needed to be conducted was complete. Early on, my siblings and I were instructed how to take proper professional business messages in my father's absence.

Growing up during the Great Depression had left an indelible mark on my father's persona. He was a successful self-made man who did everything he could to outrun the memories of the relative poverty he experienced in his family of origin, living in an apartment over a movie theatre in Cedarhurst on Long Island's south shore. His father had died when my father was seventeen and he saw it as his responsibility to drill the importance of personal responsibility into his children.

Materially, we always had what we needed, but anything we wanted beyond my father's definition of "necessary" involved doing extra chores to make the money to pay for it. When I was eleven and wanted my first pair of high quality leather basketball sneakers, I had to earn the money to pay the difference between the $9.00 cost of canvas Converse and the $16.00 Adidas Superstars that I coveted (at the time, only Adidas and Puma made high-end hoops shoes).

My mother grew up in the itty-bitty town of Oxford in the southeastern corner of Pennsylvania, about ninety minutes southwest of Philadelphia and in close proximity to Kennett Square, the self-titled "mushroom capital of the world." It was the epitome of small town life in Middle America where everyone knew everyone, and the Police Department, as my father described it, was a "hellava nice guy." My mother's otherwise typical upbringing contained the bizarre experience of sleeping in a crib from the time she was an infant until the age of seven. As she would joke, who knows how long she might have been stuck in that crib if her younger sister hadn't come along seven years to the day after my mother was born to supplant her.

Stay-at-home moms were the norm, and with the four of us my mother had a very full-time gig. She was a combination homemaker and chauffeur, shuttling us around to a wide array of activities in the family station wagon. Still, during my childhood it wasn't unusual for my mother to spend hours at a time in bed grappling with her own chronic pain and/or resting, with the aid of prescription painkillers and tranquillizers.

Ours was a liberal, progressive Jewish family, where great trust was placed in the omniscience of the medical establishment, education was prized, expectations for academic achievement and athletic performance were sky-high and without respite, and guilt was wielded like a weapon. My father routinely drilled me and my brother and sisters in various forms of mental gymnastics. When we were all together, these experiences often resembled group interviews and included all manner of subjects. The ability to respond intelligently and articulately was applauded, with extra credit given for the clever deployment of puns and double entendres. These exercises proved an excellent and occasionally ego-deflating training ground for cognitive quickness and verbal alacrity. Often they contained elements of fun, but they were nonetheless competitions and we all played to win.

Regardless of what's presented to the outside world, every family has challenges; its own gestalt of craziness and dysfunction on a continuum that can range from the stuff of nightmares and flashbacks to normative hurts that can still cut deeply and leave nasty scars. To paraphrase a comedian I've known personally since my adolescence: normal families are families we simply don't know that well.

Mine was a normal dysfunctional family. The too-close-for-comfort birth sequencing among my siblings and I made for limited psychological space to accommodate competing developmental needs, creating an extremely intense and emotionally crowded environment. There was nothing approximating the sorts of horrific, post-traumatic stress-inducing abuse that children in too many families are subjected to. Just the more usual wounds to the spirit so common in many families where parents are doing the best they can with what they have at any given moment.

Corporal punishment was a primary parenting option when I was growing up, and it was employed intermittently in our family. After getting slapped across the face for one willful indiscretion or another I found it hard to not cry. Sometimes there was a time delay after I got hit, and it was only after I thought about being smacked in the face that tears appeared. From a very young age I had a rudimentary awareness that I wasn't crying because it hurt physically; it was about the emotional injury. Those slaps to the face somehow represented a diminution of me as a person—it was a serrated affront to my psyche, and that hurt seemed bottomless.

By early elementary school, unconsciously, I had already begun to practice the art of living a double life. At home I was an oppositional-defiant hellion. Fueled by a reservoir of anger, I broke or just ignored most of the rules my parents tried to establish. And yet, whenever I went to a friend's house to visit or for a sleepover, the hosting parents would report what a polite and well-behaved child I was, leaving my own parents wondering, "Who the hell are they talking about? They must have Danny confused with someone else!" This occurred time and again. Occasionally my parents would express their frustration and confusion aloud to me, though neither they nor I had any answers.

Family systems theory views families in their entirety as an organism. Families form systems or entities that are much more than the individuals who comprise them. Every family has its own rhythm and flow, and family members develop particular ways of acting and reacting with each other and with the outside world. These specific patterns of interaction between family members give each family system a particular equilibrium and style related to such areas as expectations (spoken and unspoken); how feelings are expressed (or not); how conflict is managed (or avoided); how family issues are communicated in the world outside the family system; and what roles and responsibilities family members are assigned—consciously and unconsciously. These dynamics shape the personality styles and behaviors of each family member.

Change in *any* part of the system creates ripple-effect changes in *all* parts of the system. Think of a mobile hanging from the ceiling in a child's room: when one part moves, all of the other parts move in response to it. When one family member is overly responsible and controlling, this shapes the behaviors of other family members. They typically respond by becoming somewhat less responsible. The equilibrium of the family system shifts as each member changes and adjusts accordingly. When a parent struggles with chronic pain (or addiction or any other serious chronic condition), his or her parenting is affected.

Virgina Satir was a social worker and psychotherapist who was a seminal figure in the developing field of family therapy in the late 1950s and early 1960s. Her original work regarding family roles was adapted by Claudia Black and Sharon Wegscheider-Cruse in the 1980s to describe the roles taken on by children in dysfunctional family systems. The framework they developed applies to many families, but especially those wrestling with momentous challenges such as addiction, trauma, physical and/or emotional violence, depression and other forms of psychiatric illness, physical and developmental disabilities, and chronic pain or serious physical illness.

These roles and their related behaviors represent unconscious psychological survival strategies that children use in order to cope with the stresses within their family. While each child in the family generally assumes a primary role, the roles themselves are far from set in cement. Family members can take on aspects of different roles, or migrate from one role to another over time and psychosocial stage of development. These roles are attempts to bring greater consistency, structure, and emotional safety into family systems that are experienced as unpredictable, chaotic, or frightening. They include, Hero, Lost Child, Mascot, and Scapegoat.

The *Hero* is the hyper-responsible child present in virtually every dysfunctional family. Usually, though not always, the hero is the oldest child. Children who assume this role are high achievers, getting excellent grades in school and excelling in sports and/or other extracurricular activities. Their behavior is exemplary—they comply with the rules and provide a model that parents, teachers, and coaches wish others would follow. Accordingly, the Hero elicits outsized approval and praise from both parents and outsiders. The family Hero reduces tension in the family simply by doing everything "right" and deflecting attention away from the family's challenges.

The *Lost Child* generally comes from the middle of the birth order, surrounded by older and younger siblings. This role is defined by the absence of a distinct role within the family system. Lost children avoid bringing attention to themselves, preferring to stay below the family radar. They often isolate, withdrawing from family and social activities to escape, and tend to distance themselves emotionally through immersion in television, computers, video games, or reading. Family members tend not to worry much about this child because he or she is quiet and appears content. As a result, it's not unusual for family members not to notice that the child isn't participating and seems withdrawn or even depressed.

The *Mascot* is almost always one of the youngest children in the family, and most frequently is the youngest. The Mascot's function is to be cute and humorous. By being cute, adorable, and/or funny they protect themselves from negative attention and distract others from the stress and dysfunction in the family. Since the Mascot tends to be the youngest, the family usually views the child with that role as the most fragile and vulnerable, and tends to be especially protective toward him or her.

The *Scapegoat* role is usually adopted by a middle child, often the second oldest. The Scapegoat is the antithesis of the Hero; the designated black sheep of the family. Who did it (whatever "it" is)? Chances are, it was the family Scapegoat. And chances are even better that the Scapegoat will be blamed for it, even if he or she didn't do it. The Scapegoat's role is to divert attention away from family's systemic dysfunction by acting out in ways that draw significant negative attention to him or her individually. In doing so, the Scapegoat unconsciously concretizes the family's problems and accepts the blame for them, while simultaneously giving expression to the family's frustration and upset.

The Scapegoat's acting out can take manifold forms, such as marked oppositionalism and rebelliousness against authority at home, in school, and/or in the community; poor academic performance; aggressive or violent behavior; and involvement in thrill-seeking or other high-risk and potentially self-destructive activities. Not surprisingly, the Scapegoat is the child most likely to have problems related to truancy, school suspensions or expulsions, arrests, sexual promiscuity, teen pregnancy, and substance use/abuse. Usually, the Scapegoat's angry, defiant, "Fuck you, I don't give a shit" outward appearance masks considerable pain. This child is frequently the most emotional and sensitive, though he or she has learned to fend off inadequacy, hurt, and rejection by employing defense mechanisms that keep these feelings of vulnerability at a safer distance.

There was never any competition for the role of Scapegoat in my family—I monopolized that designation. I was *the* "bad" kid. The two literal messages from my parents that resonated the loudest throughout my childhood were, "You're not living up to your potential," and "It's your responsibility to be a good role model for your brother and sisters." On their face, these messages were neither problematic nor unhealthy. They reflected my parents' concern and sincere desire for me to excel and to be the best person I could be. But they also reinforced the pressure of certain unrelenting expectations and the assessment that I was failing to meet them.

The impact of words is always influenced by the accompanying nonverbal cues of facial expression, tone of voice, and body language. The emotional tone with which such messages are communicated makes a massive difference in the meanings they convey. The emotional tone of the above messages to me was sometimes of frustration or anger, but always of disappointment. The effect was shaming, and the embedded meanings I internalized were that I wasn't good enough and that I wasn't enough.

From an early age, I exhibited a hyper-sensitivity to emotions. I experienced feelings such as hurt, sadness, guilt, shame, and anger with heightened acuity, seemingly more rapidly and deeply than most other people. This set off a tuning-fork-like reactivity and a long-term affair with anger. Anger was like an ever-present low-lying fog limiting my visibility. From the time I began to experience that the world sometimes ignored my desires and perceived needs, anger was always there for me—convincing me that I was getting screwed, fueling my self-righteous emotional escalation and acting out. During my MSW program I would learn that in children and adolescents, pervasive anger is often a symptom of depression.

In sixth grade CYO basketball (though Jewish, I played in a Catholic Youth Organization league because that's where the best competition was), my coach put into words something that I already knew well: "The best defense is a good offense; if we have the ball, they cannot score!" This described the essence of my approach, not only to basketball and other sports, but also to coping with all manner of uncomfortable emotions and situations. In terms of emotions and their expression, anger is the most potent embodiment of "the best defense is a good offense."

In the vast majority of circumstances, anger is a secondary emotion, forming almost immediately and automatically in response to someone or something that brings up feelings of hurt, fear, shame, and inadequacy or of not being good-enough. These primary emotions made me feel weak and vulnerable—self-perceptions that were intolerable to me as a child. I used anger as a defense against them, a shield that deflected them and gave me power. Anger like this serves two important psychological purposes: it provides a sense of control when one is desperately needed, and it directs our focus outward, providing identifiable, external others, indeed, scapegoats, to blame.

Displacement is a defense mechanism that unconsciously transfers unacceptable thoughts, feelings, or desires from a psychologically unsafe object to a more acceptable, less threatening substitute. A classic example is the man who is angry at his boss and cannot express it directly so he comes home and kicks the family dog or yells at his wife and kids. When we cannot confront the real sources of our anger, hurt, fear, and pain because they hold power over us, we tend to take it out on someone who is weaker and effectively "safer." Children engage in displacement when it is too anxiety-provoking to consciously acknowledge and express upset at parents and other caregivers they are dependent upon for their survival needs. Instead, they tease the cat, bully someone at school, or lash out at younger siblings.

Although there were many times when we had fun and played together, my brother and sisters were safe objects onto which my anger was regularly displaced. I treated them so badly. I could be mean to the point of cruelty. I'd call them names and put them down verbally. Occasionally I'd hit them, usually in the big muscles of the biceps and thighs, giving them "dead" arms and legs. While the physical abuse I perpetrated was sporadic, to them the implied threat of it was constant, and the emotional abuse ongoing. I've come to learn that when we were left alone at home they consistently felt unsafe, because of me. It wasn't unusual for them to lock themselves behind closed doors, hoping I wouldn't find a way to break in, though often I did.

My anger was generalized and free-floating, always searching for concrete targets to latch onto. Most of the time I wasn't consciously aware of how angry I was, or even what it was that I was angry about. And during our formative years, my siblings bore the brunt of it as I terrorized them. A vicious circle ensued wherein my parents would get angry at my behavior and punish me, and I'd feel that much more rejected and angry, taking it out on my brother and sisters, which only elicited more anger from my parents. As absorbed as I was in acting out my anger, there was no space left for me to appreciate that my siblings were being traumatized.

I lied like a rug, though sometimes it was blended with degrees of denial and a child's magical thinking that if I didn't admit to it, the reality would just go away. I shaded the truth and told half-lies or lies of omission, and sometimes I was straight up dishonest. I lied to make myself look better. I lied to try to feel better about myself. At times I lied for reasons outside my conscious awareness. Most often I lied to evade the consequences of my behavior. I became so used to lying that I lied even when it would have been just as easy to tell the truth.

I lied so frequently that I lost credibility for telling the truth and became like the boy who cried wolf. My parents were so accustomed to me lying that they assumed I was, even when I was telling the truth. Of course, this only exacerbated my feelings of rejection and emotional abandonment, and provided another source for my anger. My younger brother (the family Hero) learned that he could do something wrong and lie about it, confident I would catch the blame and that our parents would believe him rather than me.

As practiced as I was, I never perfected the art of lying. I was basically a shitty liar, unable to separate my internal responses from my external presentation. Inside, I knew it was wrong and part of me felt guilty. This discomfort expressed itself through my body language, and those who knew me best usually could identify my prevarications.

Anger triggered my ardent oppositionalism and rebelliousness. Overt at home, it was more subtle and indirect at school. I was an inveterate wise-ass and unrepentant class-clown. In third grade my class-clowning incited the teacher to try to hit me (this was an era that allowed public school teachers to discipline students physically with relative impunity; one teacher who some of my friends had the misfortune of having was renowned for picking kids up by their hair). I ducked and she missed, striking her hand hard on my desk before sending me to the principal's office where I was well acquainted with the office staff. Most of the office staff wondered how a student as polite and well-mannered as me could get in as much trouble as I seemed to. My parents only wanted to know what I had done to provoke the teacher, assuming that I had deserved her wrath. Fourth grade marked the first of many times when I got in trouble for using profanity in school.

My acting out brought me to Dr. Seymour Gruber, a child psychiatrist in Great Neck, NY (actually, it was my mother who brought me to the good doctor). By this time, my parents figured there was a real problem, and it was me. Appointments with Dr. Gruber got me out of school early and sessions were painless enough, spent making model ships and airplanes while talking about whatever. Still, it reinforced the feelings I had of being different and damaged. He diagnosed some sort of nonspecific chemical imbalance and put me on Dilantin, a medication typically used to manage epilepsy and other seizure disorders. Though not FDA-approved for it, there are indications that Dilantin can be helpful in stabilizing mood and managing anxiety, and it's sometimes prescribed "off label" for those purposes.

Interestingly, Dilantin was used both as an anticonvulsant and as a chemical restraint to control patient behavior in *One Flew Over the Cuckoo's Nest*, Ken Kesey's acclaimed novel about a locked psychiatric facility and the interactions between the milieu and its unfortunate inhabitants. Of course, Kesey's main character was a recalcitrant rebel rather than someone suffering from severe mental illness, but that didn't keep him from being lobotomized.

Throughout elementary school my grades were mostly "A"s with a small smattering of "B"s. "B"s were cause for questions and concerns at home. In fifth grade, I got a "C" in math one marking period and based on my parents' reactions, a casual observer might have thought there was a death in the family. My siblings routinely produced straight "A"s. They did their schoolwork with dedication and consistency, whereas my approach gravitated toward getting the best grades I could while doing as little actual work as possible.

Thank god for sports. Sports were my safe haven and my saving grace. It was the one area of life where I felt whole and good enough. The athletic arena—whether a baseball diamond, football field, basketball court, or lacrosse field—provided an environment where I had a coherent sense of self and a clear sense of self-worth. It didn't matter whether it was a school yard pickup game or formal league play, I was given freedom from the feeling that I was a fuck-up. There was something transcendent in how sports integrated my body and mind. The hand-eye coordination required to track and catch a deep pass in football, to time and hit a baseball on the fat part of the bat, or to gauge the distance to the rim and execute the proper trajectory to make an outside shot in basketball had a present-centered life-affirming melody all its own. To me, these were majestic pursuits, and when I was immersed in them, the dis-ease that followed me wherever I went for as long as I could remember melted away.

Although I was always drawn toward team sports, I busted my ass to hone my individual skills, practicing constantly, pushing myself to get better: shooting baskets on an outdoor court covered in snow and ice in the dead of winter; playing catch until it was too dark to see even the outline of the baseball or football against the evening sky; coming early to team practices and staying late. When I was nine, I remember committing to myself to continue playing after basketball practice until I had made 100 additional baskets. It didn't matter how long it was going to take; I was staying until I accomplished that goal or they kicked me out of the gym.

In spite of the occasional intrusion of interpersonal politics in the form of favoritism, nepotism, or cliques, sports represented a meritocracy where you got what you earned. Schoolyard pickup games (regardless of sport) had a well-defined social order. The acknowledged two best players were designated captains who took turns choosing players for their respective teams from among the assembled kids. There was a direct correlation between your skills and when you were selected—the better you were, the sooner you were picked. I could count on one hand the number of times I wasn't either a captain or among the first players picked. This selection process was fraught with emotion. As it progressed, with each successive selection, I watched the facial expressions of many kids fall as their hope to be picked earlier faded. If there were more kids than available places on the teams, some didn't get to play at all. I always felt the anguish of those who were picked toward the end or not at all; of those who were not good enough.

Sports provided an ideal sublimation for my anger. Sublimation is a more "healthy" defense mechanism that channels or redirects unacceptable thoughts, feelings, and urges, into socially acceptable pursuits. It takes the energy of something potentially harmful and turns it to a constructive and useful activity. Athletic competition was a socially acceptable and emotionally safe outlet to discharge my energy and emotion, especially anger. Instead of criticism, feelings of inadequacy, and punitive consequences, as long as I could convert my anger and other heated emotions into sports-related competitive fervor, I experienced feelings of achievement and received positive recognition and high praise. In this context, I knew who I was and that I was worthy.

The only downside of this passion for sports was its ignition of a white-hot competitiveness that combined with rapacious perfectionism to drive me to be too hard on teammates, oppressive to referees and umpires (I set a record for technical fouls in Oyster Bay youth basketball in the early 1970s that probably still stands), and merciless toward myself. However, were it not for competitive sports and the cathartic release they provided,

I have little doubt that I would have become part of the juvenile justice and/or youth psychiatric systems at a tender age.

My involvement in sports was also a sanctuary from much of the tension and conflict between my parents and me. In this special sphere, my parents were consistently available for me. They were models of emotional and practical support. Despite his nonstop work schedule, my father somehow still made time to play catch with me; throw pitches to me so I could practice batting and learn how to switch-hit; throw passes to me on the run until being able to touch the football meant I would catch it; and shoot hoops and play one-on-one with me on the court in our driveway—for what seemed like hours at a time. My mother drove me to and picked me up from hundreds of practices, often giving rides to my friends and teammates who didn't have parents willing or able to be there like that for them. When I earned the money to get those $16.00 Adidas, she drove me across the width of Long Island to Wolf's Sporting Goods in Rockeville Centre, the only store on Long Island that carried them.

My parents were a constant presence in the bleachers and on the sidelines at my games from little league to high school, regardless of the sport. My father's expectations for performance were evident in his urgent and high-volume exhortations to me and his vehement critiques of the officiating, which could always easily be heard above the din of the game and other crowd noise. At times it was so obtrusive and embarrassing that in the midst of playing I'd yell at him to stop. On at least one occasion the referees kicked him out of the gym altogether. My father offered to coach my teams in youth sports, but given how conflicted our relationship often was, I didn't want him to. When he later coached some of my younger brother's teams, I remember feeling a mix of relief, envy, and sadness.

That ambivalence hit the heart of the relationship I had with my parents. There were many instances when they were available and nurturing, and yet, overall, I felt emotionally rejected and abandoned. Although I had an abstract cognizance that they loved me, the impression that they didn't like me was tangible.

Besides carting my siblings and I around like a car service, my mother spent many hours helping me with school projects in elementary school. She was also my very first writing teacher. I've been calling her by her first name since I was in seventh grade. One day I started doing it and she allowed it so I kept doing it, and it became normal. Though my friends always thought this was strange, I never gave it much thought until I was thirty-one years old and happened to mention it during an individual therapy session with Bob, an exceptionally wise and skillful psychotherapist. He was struck by the dynamics inherent in my calling my mother by her first name from such an unusually young age and offered an interpretation: beneath the surface of my conscious awareness I had concluded that in order to feel safer psychologically I needed to put more emotional distance between my mother and me, and calling her by her first name served that purpose. As I reflected in silence on Bob's hypothesis, its ring of truth grew louder.

There is no way to know whether my incipient acting out precipitated my parents' judgment of me as the "problem" child, or whether my early unconscious perceptions that I wasn't good enough for them spurred my anger and acting out. These family dynamics evolved dialectically, each influencing the other directly and indirectly, until both of them became "true." Like all self-fulfilling prophesies, this scenario was the product of an interaction between beliefs and behaviors, wherein how a situation or person is characterized evokes attitudes and actions, which bring that characterization to fruition. Like a snowball rolling downhill, as the process continues, it gathers speed and momentum, going faster and becoming harder to stop.

chapter three

[THROUGH THE LOOKING GLASS]

"It takes dynamite to get me up
Too much of everything is just enough"
JOHN BARLOW, *I NEED A MIRACLE,* GRATEFUL DEAD

Everyone has a certain personality style that includes core traits. When these constitutionally endowed qualities combine with the roles we adapt in our family system, it contorts the lens through which we see ourselves and we get a distorted view of who we are. This misshapen self-perception impacts how we relate to ourselves, to others, and to the world.

We learn to view ourselves in a way that mirrors how others seem to view and treat us. Unconditional positive regard refers to the elemental acceptance and emotional support of a person regardless of what he or she may say or do. It describes the simple but potent actions, in words, attitudes, and deeds, of accepting someone for who he or she truly is—with all of his or her mistakes and imperfections. Carl Rogers, the founder of Client-Centered Therapy—a humanistic approach that undergirds many contemporary forms of counseling and psychotherapy—considered unconditional positive regard requisite to healthy psychological development and made the therapeutic application of it a cornerstone of his model of helping people.

For most of us, the acceptance and positive regard granted us by others has been conditional. In other words, they are commonly attached to various conditions of "worth." Growing up we were shown acceptance and positive regard when we demonstrated that we were somehow "worthy," rather than unconditionally because we deserved it simply by virtue of our humanity. Many of us have had the experience of getting positive attention, acceptance, affection, and love if, and sometimes only if, we behaved to the satisfaction of others.

Because we have natural human needs for acceptance and positive regard, the conditions under which they are given exert a persuasive influence. We tend to mold ourselves into shapes determined by family and social expectations—expectations that may or may not align with our best interests. Over time, this results in conditional positive self-regard/self-esteem, where we may like or even accept ourselves only if we meet the standards others have applied to us. And since these standards are generally disconnected from our individual needs and differences, often we find ourselves unable to meet them or unwilling to accommodate them, and in turn, unable to maintain a coherent sense of self-worth.

Having to hide a part of oneself in order to be accepted and considered good enough on a consistent basis is a form of emotional rejection and abandonment. D. W. Winnicott was a British pediatrician turned psychoanalyst who wrote extensively about this process and how it can affect the way people relate to themselves and others. According to Winnicott, the need to effectively dance to the tunes of others, especially primary caregivers early in life—in denying our own genuine individual needs—obstructs the development of a healthy and congruent "true self," and results in the formation of a "false self."

The false self can be compliant, reacting to environmental demands by accepting them willingly and uncritically, or rebellious, opposing, and aggressively rejecting those demands. In either of these configurations, a false self creates an inauthentic set of relationships, even though they have every appearance of being real. Because this is a wholly unconscious process, the false self comes to be mistaken for the true self by others, and even by oneself. Although this false self persona serves a useful defensive purpose, it becomes an enduring mask, obscuring our real nature and creating considerable internal conflict (often underneath the surface of conscious awareness). It can also greatly increase one's vulnerability to the significant psychosocial problems. Did someone say addiction?

I was in fifth grade when the Nassau County police visited Vernon Elementary School, going classroom to classroom with a large display case filled with different types of drugs, all neatly laid out and labeled. We were treated to all of the horror stories steeped in the zeitgeist of the late 1960s. I promised myself that day I would NEVER do drugs—any of them. Bit by bit and substance by substance that promise—which I absolutely meant at the time—disintegrated. I started drinking toward the end of sixth grade, rationalizing that alcohol was different, and that I wouldn't ever use "drugs." By seventh grade I was smoking pot.

However risk-laden the path I was on might have been already, seventh grade marked a turning point into darker territory. The three local elementary schools fed into Oyster Bay Junior High School, which placed students in one of four levels based on a combination of grades and standardized test scores. "Honors" was the top of the line, for the brightest kids; "College" was the designation for those considered above average; average students were placed in "Regents," and then there was a level for kids who were assessed as being below average. It was a curious form of academic segregation—students attended classes almost exclusively within their designated level.

There were approximately three hundred kids in our seventh grade, and only seventeen of us were placed in Honors. I found myself in the midst of the nerdiest, geekiest kids in the entire grade. Even though some of them were friends from elementary school, and as a group they were certainly nice enough, I was in shock; surely there had been a mistake—I didn't belong there! Most of my close friends were placed in Regents, with a few in College. My sense of being different and of not fitting in discovered a new source of nourishment.

I spent the school year proving to myself and everyone else that I wasn't like my brainiac classmates, culminating with getting caught in possession of a Scotch-filled water pistol. I created enough havoc that at the conclusion of the school year I was "invited" to leave the public school system—an exceedingly rare occurrence in 1972.

In eighth grade I became acquainted with pills, notably barbiturates. It was also during eighth grade that I was introduced to the wonderful world of opioids, by my mother. We had gone to visit my aunt and uncle for a long holiday weekend when I came down with a skull-imploding headache. Over-the-counter pain relievers had no effect. The pain was so searing and unremitting that my mother decided to give me half a Percodan. As the adults left to go out for the evening, she left the prescription bottle on the night stand next to me with instructions that if the pain didn't get better I could take another half a pill.

I was still in the infancy of my drug use, but I knew enough to know that if half a pill could be helpful, than a whole one would be better, so that's what I took. I just wanted the pain to stop and the first half I had taken hadn't done shit. After what seemed like a few short minutes, my pain dissolved and I was submerged in a luscious, warm, radiant nirvana. I marveled at how delicious it felt. It felt like how I had always wanted to feel.

One of the variables that correlates with the potential for addiction is how someone reacts to the effects of drugs. Research has shown that those who have negative reactions, such as nausea, dizziness, or confusion, are at lower risk for addiction. Those who have more positive reactions, like euphoria, anxiety reduction, or increased energy, are at higher risk.

Somewhere around this time, during a visit to my maternal grandparents in Pennsylvania, my grandmother gave me a laminated wallet-sized card, saying "I want you to have this." On it in beautiful calligraphy the following words were inscribed: *God grant me the Serenity to accept the things I cannot change; the Courage to change the things I can, and the Wisdom to know the difference*—the Serenity Prayer. The very first time I read those words they had immediate heft and resonance, as well as an inchoate soothing effect. As I looked at the card and read the words again, my breathing became a little deeper and my pulse rate slowed slightly. I may not have been able to grasp the magnitude of their simple and elegant wisdom, but even then I knew the message they carried was important.

My maternal grandparents were steadfast in their support for me. They were the closest thing to unconditional love and acceptance I knew. They were always in my corner—even when I was a complete asshole to my grandmother, as I was on multiple occasions as a teenager. As the eldest grandson, "grandson number one" as he would say, I held a special place in my grandfather's heart. The two of us were the only avid bowlers in the family. Although he hadn't bowled in years due to a bad back, whenever I visited, he would take to the local lanes, watch me bowl, and give me pointers.

In ninth and tenth grades I played JV basketball and varsity lacrosse at Long Island Lutheran High School, which was close by and perennially had among the top high school basketball teams in the state. Their teams regularly included some of the most talented players from New York City, who lived with local families during the school year. The varsity coach's favorite saying: "Practice doesn't make perfect. Only perfect practice makes perfect." The skill-development training in this program was cutting-edge—the drills we practiced and the techniques we honed through countless repetitions would not become mainstream until years later.

The JV and the varsity basketball teams often worked out together. The practices were brutal and the competition fierce. One of the best ways to get better—at anything—is to play with and against people who are better than you are. I was long used to being among the shortest players on the court (unfortunately you can't "learn" height), but now I was going up against players who were not only much bigger, but whose athleticism was astonishing. Every day I had to play my ass off just to hold my own. I established a niche through hustle play that included sacrificing my body: diving on the court for loose balls and on defense, stepping directly in front of an oncoming opposing player and allowing him to effectively run me over, creating an offensive foul and giving my team the ball. I learned how to fall in ways that minimized the impacts to my body, but the long-term consequences of hundreds of collisions with other players and between my back and the hardwood would later exact its toll.

Sometimes I played with more balls than brains. Once in practice, the varsity center had the ball on a fast break. He was 6'8", 235 pounds, first team All-New York State, and on this occasion, moving at high speed, focused on the rim, and getting ready to throw down a monster slam dunk, when I (over a foot shorter and 100 pounds lighter) positioned myself directly in his path to take a charge. He was a close friend of mine, and off the court, a proverbial gentle giant. When he saw that I wasn't going to move, his eyes filled with "Are you outta your motherfuckin'mind!!" alarm. In his split-second attempt to avoid colliding with—and possibly permanently damaging—me, he lost his balance and committed a traveling violation. It may have been an episode of situation-specific insanity where I put myself quite literally in harm's way, but it turned a certain two points into a turnover and gave my team the ball. It was also just one of many instances where I would place myself in positions of high risk for momentary reward.

When I got to high school, I made a conscious decision to try "everything" in terms of mind- and mood-altering substances, and to try enough of each to make an informed decision as to what I liked and wanted to use more of. Though I didn't get high on days I had practice or games (at least until after the practice or game), overall my drug use continued to progress. I returned to public school in eleventh grade after the new varsity basketball coach at Oyster Bay High School (who had been my lacrosse coach at Lutheran) encouraged me to come play for him. A season of great promise short-circuited when I tore a quadriceps muscle in my left thigh toward the end of an otherwise excellent first game. That injury sidelined me for most of the rest of the season while I went through physical therapy and wallowed in frustration and disappointment as I watched the team play from the far-off distance of the bench.

As much as I was in love with playing, as good as I was, as hard as I worked at it, the levels of physicality and ability I encountered while at Lutheran brought home the limitations of my "upside." The realization that my participation in sports would never be more than an avocation was a huge and painful loss. As my childhood dream of getting paid to play hoops died, I lost the only real motivation I had for not using, and jumped the line that separates steady recreational substance use from full-on addiction.

I dove headlong into applied neurochemistry, that is, learning through intensive first-hand experiential study how the full spectrum of drugs—alone and in myriad combinations—affected me, as well as how adjustments in dosage modified those effects. I became adept in medicine cabinet archeology, a related discipline that involved exploring and excavating the contents of medicine cabinets wherever I went in order to unearth materials to further my neurochemical studies. Rather than treating my body as a temple, I increasingly used it as an amusement park.

I had started going to bars with older friends shortly after I turned fifteen. At the time, the drinking age was eighteen and it was easy to use other people's identification as New York state driver's licenses didn't yet have pictures. Shit, they didn't even indicate hair color—for a time I used the ID of a friend who had bright red hair. Pot was ever-present, like paint on the walls, and I remained under its influence as much as I could.

I contrasted the consciousness-expanding exhilaration of LSD with the consciousness-contracting confines of PCP. PCP outfitted me with a perceptual straitjacket, requiring a half-hour to crawl up a flight of stairs. Dozens of acid trips blew open the doors to new universes and let me borrow the keys to some of the mysteries of this one. By the way, taking LSD while at school is a really bad idea—that's why I did it twice.

My way of identifying where the limits—both internal and external—were, was to exceed them, leaving them in the dust . . . repeatedly. As my father put it during one of my blood-shot mornings after another night of debauchery, "Moderation Dan, look it up!" I stole hundreds of pills from my mother. I took so many that I knew that she knew, but nothing was said. We engaged in an unacknowledged dance: she kept finding new hiding places for her meds, and I kept finding them. When we finally talked about it in shared sadness, I said, "I kept waiting for you to say something," to which she replied, "I kept waiting for you to stop."

Adding the self-centeredness of active addiction to the developmentally based narcissism of adolescence makes for a noxious combination. The relationship between my parents and me deteriorated, becoming more overtly conflicted as I increasingly disrespected them and their authority and ignored any limits they attempted to set. It got to the point where my father and I couldn't be in the same room together for more than a few minutes before an argument would ignite and escalate until he would come after me physically, chasing me out of the room and out of the house. I would return hours later.

As this pattern continued, I began to stay away from home overnight, and then for several days at a time. The mounting tension finally exploded altogether when my father and I got in the one and only physical fight we've ever had. I had a furious argument with my mother and threw a football hard in her direction, hitting her in the foot. I didn't think that I wanted to hit her, but I could have made sure to avoid it. When my father came home and learned what happened, he understandably flew into a rage and came after me. This time I didn't run. It only lasted a few minutes, no punches were thrown, and there were no physical injuries, but for me it was terrifying and traumatic. I left the house fighting back tears and totally freaked out, knowing that it would be a long time before I could return.

I was able to stay with a family I knew well, whose two daughters were among my close friends. To my relief and my parents' surprise, they generously allowed me to live with them from August through December of 1976. During that time I was introduced to two new areas that would open my eyes in unexpected ways. Faye, the mother in the family with whom I stayed, was the first person to teach me about consciousness—how our mind determines to a great extent our relationship with ourselves, with others, and with the world; and how so much of our subjective experience is a function of our perception. For the first time, I began to get a sense of the spiritual as distinct from the religious, as well as understand drug-induced states of consciousness as part of a much larger continuum.

The physical separation from my parents gave us all room to breathe. The distance allowed us the space for a gradual rapprochement, and after about a month I started to have dinner with my family once a week. At my parents' urging, we also began family therapy. I didn't want to participate in family therapy and I was convinced that it would be a waste of time, but I also didn't want to bear the weight of responsibility for not being willing to try since so many of the family's problems seemed to track back to me. Moreover, I really did want to have a relationship with my family and had no idea how to get there from where we were.

Family therapy was both challenging and fascinating. Our therapist was an experienced and savvy MSW who used an explicitly family systems approach. Even though—as is so often the case with the Scapegoat—it was my acting out that brought the family into therapy, to my amazement I was not blamed. As much focus was placed on my parents and on my siblings as on me. As uncomfortable as I know it was for my parents, particularly for my father, to not be in charge, they were open and receptive. Family therapy changed how we related to one another, and for a time, communication within our family, and between my parents and me, improved dramatically.

All through this period, I continued to develop my capacity to live a double life, negotiating very different worlds—precariously balancing a "B"+ average with the roles of druggie, varsity athlete, pot dealer, and student council vice president. My group of close friends dubbed me "Citizen Dan" for my ability to shift gears and strap on a diplomatic persona whenever it served my purposes.

I moved back home in early January 1977, and having accumulated enough credits to graduate early, completed high school later that month. I graduated somewhere toward the bottom of the top 15 percent of my class. Some family context: my brother would become valedictorian, graduating first in his high school class; one of my sisters was salutatorian, graduating second in her class; and my other sister graduated somewhere between the top 5 and 10 percent of her class. When I said good-bye to high school, I was well versed in the three "R"s (well, not so much 'rithmetic—math and I never got along well) and intimately familiar with the four "S"s—smoking, swallowing, snorting, and shooting.

Two weeks later, at the age of seventeen, I left New York and most everything that was familiar to me 3,000 miles behind. I had spent a month during the previous summer hitchhiking around California with a friend, and decided then to attend college there. With a one-way plane ticket and $200.00 in my pocket, I moved to Los Angeles by myself, forsaking the glory days of my senior year of high school to work full-time and get a head start on establishing state residency prior to beginning school at the University of California at Santa Cruz that fall.

At the time, I knew one person in LA, an uncle who had had a nasty divorce from my aunt ten years earlier, whom I had visited briefly during the previous summer. I lived at his home in Downey for the first month, which also coincided with my first job as an independent adult—selling encyclopedias door-to-door. As bad as that gig was, from it came an unexpected benefit. I became friends with a coworker who had a friend with a small house in Temple City who needed a roommate. For the following eight months I shacked up with Perry, who despite being legally blind rode a motorcycle and somehow had a legitimate California state motorcycle license. I got a job at a glass manufacturing company in East LA, which required taking two different buses, over an hour each way, to get to and from work. Although I used daily, my LA experience gave me important opportunities to grow up and provided a less-than-appetizing taste of what the adult world of work can mean, reinforcing my appreciation for higher education.

The University of California at Santa Cruz is a singular place—2,000 acres of redwood-covered forest, interspersed with wide meadows overlooking the Pacific Ocean and the city of Santa Cruz with its stunning beaches, stretches of sand extending between cliffs perched on the northern tip of Monterey Bay. Established by the University of California as an "alternative" campus in 1965, it was unique in combining the resources and prestige of a major university with the intimate feel of a small, liberal arts college and a rigorous academic environment. After exerting so little effort in school, I was finally ready to invest myself academically.

Even still, throughout my tenure at UC Santa Cruz, I walked a tightrope between working hard and performing well academically and pursuing pleasure pharmacologically. I lived on campus my freshman year and my dorm was located next to some administrative offices. On one occasion, an office assistant followed the pungent aroma of pot to my room and politely requested that I find a way to keep the smoke from infiltrating their building. It was as matter-of-fact as if she were asking me to turn down the live Grateful Dead that I routinely played at loud volume.

Wacky names for college intramural sports teams are not unusual, but during my sophomore year our intramural flag football team likely broke new ground. "The U-40s" was the brainchild of a small group of like-minded friends who shared an affinity for both sports and intravenous drug use, and may be the only intramural team ever named after a specific model of syringe.

I graduated in the spring of 1981 with a double major in Psychology and Environmental Studies/Planning and Public Policy, and an asterisk. The asterisk was that while I received my BA in Psychology with Honors, I had completed all of the requirements for my degree in Planning and Public Policy except one—an extensive senior thesis. Environmental Studies, and the degree I didn't quite yet have, was my real interest. The program at Santa Cruz was state-of-the-art; the coursework was challenging and thought-provoking, and the professors were awe-inspiring yet approachable. My psychology major was also excellent and growth-enhancing, but I added it basically as a throw-in to achieve the distinction of a double major. I had fully planned to finish my senior thesis the year following my graduation.

chapter four

[IF YOU MEET THE BUDDHA,]
SAY HELLO

"Sometimes the light's all shining on me
Other times I can barely see."
ROBERT HUNTER, *TRUCKIN'*, GRATEFUL DEAD

In October of 1981, a few months after completing one of my two degrees and going through the graduation ceremony at UC Santa Cruz, I went backpacking in Desolation Wilderness near Lake Tahoe with Mick, then one of my closest friends. Mick had graduated the year before me and was working construction at the time, even though he was a genius in science and math. He had an innate ability to understand how the world works on those levels—areas that have always been a mystery to me. Mick was also one of my hardest-core partying partners. There were frighteningly few mind- and mood-altering rocks that we hadn't turned over together to explore in-depth what was underneath.

The very first time we met, perhaps not surprisingly, revolved around drugs. I was on the prowl for pot during my first week at UCSC, looking to find, not just a place to score now, but a reliable ongoing source. A friend of a new friend directed me to the dorm next to mine, to a room at the end of the top floor, and there was Mick, wanting to know why I was there. Even though I came with my referral source who lived in that same dorm and I looked no older than my eighteen years, complete with long thick hair down to nearly the middle of my back, Mick immediately suspected that I was a cop. As much as I was tempted to respond with laughter and sarcasm, my mission was serious and I didn't want to risk leaving empty handed, so I asked what I could do to assure him that I was just a new student who wanted to get high. After satisfying him with my answers to a battery of questions, we concluded our business. It took a few months for Mick to warm up to me, but over time we developed a tight bond.

We had planned to be in the wilderness for three days, and stopped at the Safeway in South Lake Tahoe to pick up supplies. Most critically, a quality steak to go with the killer Cabernet Sauvignon that we had selected for the first evening's meal. After all, camping in the high altitude wilderness of the Sierra Nevada was no reason not to have a high class dinner. While waiting in the checkout line, I gradually became aware that several lines away the cashier seemed to be engaged, and engaging everyone who came through his line, in having an absolutely great time—on the checkout line at Safeway!

The scene was simultaneously bizarre and compelling. I found myself instantly drawn to this cashier and the quality of his interactions with customers. He was short, bald, rotund to the point of being obese, and wore thick old-school black horn-rimmed eyeglasses. He didn't just greet his customers; he embraced them: each and every one, in a verbal/

emotional bear-hug of warm, welcoming, it's-wonderful-to-see-you-again-my-old-friend energy.

His manner was boisterous to the point of standing out, yet neither obnoxious nor intrusive. It was congruent rather than contrived, as genuine and natural as the Ponderosa Pines and Douglas Fir trees dotting the landscape around Tahoe. I was mesmerized. Although I wasn't entirely certain what was going on here, I knew that it was exceedingly rare.

Somehow, in the midst of one of the more mundane, often frustrating environments on the planet, this short, bald, fat grocery store cashier seemed to be operating in a state of unadulterated joy that allowed him to appear to float ever so slightly above the ground that constrained the rest of us. There was a certain music and magic to this person and how he related to others and to the world. Whatever it was that he had, I wanted to experience it up close. I then did something I have never done in my entire life, either before or since. I actually switched lines to one with a noticeably longer wait, just so I would have the opportunity to be in personal contact with this phenomenon, whatever it was.

I waited in his checkout line with curiosity, anticipation, and (especially for me) extraordinary patience, noticing more carefully how the customers, without exception reacted to his unexpected and enthusiastic grace with bemused grins and a sense of wonder. When it was my turn, he greeted me with equal élan and a Cheshire cat smile that consumed most of my field of vision. I made direct eye contact and returned his greeting, adding "It's great to see someone who really seems to know how to enjoy life." He leaned toward me, lowered his voice slightly and chuckled, "And you know, it doesn't cost anything extra," at which point he gave me a knowing wink.

As his sense of present-centered joy washed over me, for a few brief seconds that felt much longer, it was as if everything else faded away, and in that moment, I knew everything that I would ever truly need to know—though I would quickly forget it. It would only occur to me years later, viewed through the perspective of twelve-step recovery and an enhanced sense of spirituality that this effervescent generosity of spirit stood on a foundation of love—simple, abundant, and pure.

As perfect as that moment was, of course it couldn't last. Perfection only visits us every once in a great while, and it never stays very long. Such transcendent experiences are always temporary. Whenever I try to keep them as if they are possessions, I invariably set myself up for disappointment. The most healthy and spiritual thing I can do is to recognize and appreciate these moments for what they are as opposed to focusing on what they are not and can never be.

Mick and I drove to the trail head for our initial eight-mile hike into the wilderness. It was a magnificent autumn afternoon in the High Sierra. The air was cool and crisp at our elevation of slightly over 7,400 feet, but it was sunny and very comfortable. Although it was mid-Autumn with its emerging potential for storms, there was no hint in the forecast that this glorious weather pattern wouldn't continue.

We set up camp at the edge of one of the smaller lakes south of Tahoe in the Desolation Wilderness. The collective spirit of nature and the universe seemed to be smiling amidst the majestic panorama of color and geology. We enjoyed a sumptuous supper centered around our rib-eye and Cabernet that merged seamlessly and sensuously on our palettes to create the synergy known by red wine aficionados in select circles as "chewy wine." Satiated by our meal, my close encounter with the Buddha at Safeway, and the serenity of the scenery, as well as a substantial stash of smack-down sinsemilla (high-end marijuana to the uninitiated), we slept soundly that night.

We awoke to the roof of our tent concaving in on us to within inches of our faces. Instinctively pushing the fabric up and outward, we displaced what in silhouette seemed to be a shitload of snow. Suddenly very awake, Mick and I looked at one another with the same thought, "No fucking way!" Upon unzipping the tent entrance we were greeted with more than two feet of fresh snow, all of which had fallen silently during the night, blanketing everything.

We were totally unprepared for anything like this. My heaviest clothing consisted of a sweater and an insulated sweatshirt. There was immediate wordless recognition that this was a serious and potentially dangerous situation. We knew without having to confer that the focus of our adventure had instantly shifted to simply finding our way back to the ranger station and our car safely.

To get to our campsite we had followed a well-delineated trail, the last part of which was a fairly steep downhill climb to the level topography around the lake. The depth and virginity of the snow made it a bitch just to identify where to pick up the trail to head back uphill. After an anxiety-provoking half hour of searching, assessing, and guessing where the hell the trail was and becoming increasingly cold and wet, I was starting to get scared. Fortunately, shortly thereafter, we were able to find what appeared to be the trail, though we were far from certain.

Apprehensively we ascended, making tediously slow progress until it became clear that we were on the right path. The mood on the trail back was 180 degrees from the easy-going, laugh-out-loud good time that defined our hike in. There were few words exchanged as we conserved our energy, concentrating intently on making forward progress, simply and steadily putting one foot in front of the other. As the sun rose higher, we found ourselves trudging through melting snow that became ankle-deep freezing water, negotiating the trail with the kind of intense determination achieved through practiced perseverance and tunnel-vision focus.

A sort of grim staying-in-each-moment intensity kicked in. The immediacy of our challenges crowded out all other considerations with one nagging exception: a gnawing feeling of anxiety—that lower-grade fear and worry of—what if? What if we can't make it back to the car due to any one of a half-dozen possibilities that could further bite us in the ass? Fear is almost always related to the unknown, to the uncertainty of the future and what it may have in store for us. But, as natural as such doubts were to the situation at hand, there was too much at stake to ruminate on them. Like the frigid water taking up more and more of the trail, these doubts could swirl around each step we took yet not penetrate . . . much . . . or so I needed to believe.

By the time we made it to the safe haven of the ranger station we were half-frozen, with hypothermia in close pursuit. Our feet were soaking wet and in bad and getting-worse-by-the-step condition, even though we were both equipped with high-quality hiking boots. As we immersed ourselves in the warm cocoon of the roaring fire, I exhaled a Yankee Stadium-sized sigh of relief while puzzling in amazement at how quickly and completely everything can change.

Most drugs of abuse produce intense initial sensations of pleasure. These sensations vary tremendously across different types of substances. In contrast to the relaxed calm that co-occurs with the immersive floating euphoria of opiates/opioids including heroin, cocaine produces a high characterized by a massive boost in energy, followed by feelings of power and grandiose self-confidence. When injected or smoked in its free-base form, coke produces an instantaneous rush that feels like a rocket blasting off, leaving Earth's gravity at break-neck speed—a massive high like the most ground-shaking orgasm multiplied by an exponent. I've heard some people describe it as feeling as though they are god. I was never that grandiose—for me it merely felt like caressing the face of god, as dopamine, the neurotransmitter most directly linked to the experience of pleasure, was released from the neurons in my brain in unnaturally occurring quantities, flooding every single synapse, where its reverberations thundered. In those moments of rapture, it felt like forever, but it only ever lasted a few short minutes at most.

For me, coming down from that exhilarating height was always as bad as the take off was good. As soon as the rush reached its apex and began to subside, withdrawal started to set in, followed by feelings of despondency and despair driven by the diminution in my brain's stash of dopamine. It was my own personal version of the space shuttle breaking up into pieces and slamming back to Earth. It is the simultaneous drives to recreate the ecstasy of the monumental rush and to escape the emotional death grip of the crash that churns the obsessive-compulsive need to continue to use coke. And it's a Sisyphean cluster-fuck. With each successive hit during a using session, the high gets a little lower and the low gets a little higher, as the brain's available inventory of dopamine is progressively depleted, until all that's left is depression.

Not having a clearer sense of what to do with the rest of my life, I figured that law school was a reasonable option and registered to take the LSAT (Law School Admission Test). The night before the exam I decided that I could inject coke one time—after all, it was only 7:30 p.m. By the time I quit for the night, it was 5:00 a.m. the following morning. Shockingly, I didn't do very well on the test. But I did use the experience as a learning opportunity of another sort.

I would never again shoot coke unless I had heroin or some other opiate/opioid or a benzodiazepine such as Valium as a neurochemical parachute, allowing me to float gently back to earth rather than crashing face first. Shortly thereafter, I transitioned to preferring heroin alone, though I remained open to the occasional speedball. For a year and a half, I lived like a vampire, using till the sun came up, confined to long-sleeve shirts in public even in summer. My senior thesis, and with it my Planning and Public Policy degree, went unfinished.

When I was first introduced to the *Diagnostic and Statistical Manual of Mental Disorders* in graduate school, the *DSM* was in its third edition. I was dumbfounded to learn that unlike multiple other drugs—opiates, alcohol, barbiturates, tranquillizers, etc.—there was no category for substance dependence (the then *DSM* equivalent of "addiction") for cocaine. Until the crack epidemic of the 1980s started ripping apart the lives of individuals, families, and whole communities like a Category 4 hurricane, the prevailing belief was that cocaine was psychologically, but not physically addictive (as if there was a definitive separation of mind from body that made for any meaningful difference between the two).

Anyone who had ever done an appreciable amount of the drug knew otherwise. My master's thesis (which was completed) addressed this topic, arguing for the addition of a category of "substance dependence" for cocaine in the *DSM*. It was an easy argument for me to make. When *DSM-IV* was published in 1994, it was there—professional expertise having finally caught up with hard-boiled experience.

The road from junkie to graduate student was circuitous and full of impediments, beginning with an arrest for the criminal sale of a controlled substance in January of 1983. My habits were expensive and I funded them through illicit manufacturing and sales. There is an inverse correlation between active addiction and judgment. As my addiction advanced, my judgment declined and with it, my attention to detail. Mail order was part of my business. It was a very different time and sending drugs through the mail was not that uncommon. I sent a large package to someone in New York who came recommended by a friend I had known since childhood and with whom I had done plenty of similar business. Little did I know that the person on the receiving end of this particular package was a cop.

Ironically, I had already made the decision that I needed a lifestyle transplant. I had dismantled my business infrastructure and was planning to move back to New York within the month. My relocation was expedited when the cops arrived early that morning with weapons drawn to wake me up and execute the warrant for my arrest. I had planned on driving back to New York; instead, I took a plane and had a police escort.

Between the time of my arrest and sentencing in May of that spring, I don't remember breathing much. Encased in prolonged stress and anxiety, I experienced physical symptoms of trauma, including elevated pulse rate, edginess, muscle tension, insomnia, and when I did sleep, I had nightmares. I went through the full gamut of emotional and psychological trauma symptoms: shock and disbelief, anger, irritability, sadness and hopelessness, worry and fear, difficultly concentrating, feeling disconnected and wanting to withdraw from others, along with unabating guilt, shame, and self-blame.

During my presentencing interview, I was asked whether I had a "drug problem." "No" I answered unequivocally, mobilizing my most deferential and diplomatic persona. "Sure, against my better judgment I sent a few packages as a favor to friends who had requested them, but it's not like I have a problem with using drugs myself." It was a line of denial, minimization, and bullshit similar to many I would hear years later as an addiction treatment professional.

I received "lifetime" probation, meaning that the length was indeterminate. After five years I was eligible to apply to have it terminated, but the decision would be based solely on the judge's discretion. If there was anything remotely positive that came out of my bust, it was that I had to change the course of my life; it was not an option not to.

After a couple of unsatisfying jobs in (legal) business, I came to the realization that since most of us have to spend so much of our waking time for so many years doing whatever it is we do for a living, if I wasn't fundamentally okay with my chosen vocation, I'd be setting myself up for long-term discontent. I figured that since I had a degree in psychology, I should try to put it to use.

At about the same time during the end of the summer in 1984, my girlfriend and I got married. Even though I was from Long Island and she was from northern New Jersey, we met in psychology classes at UC Santa Cruz. For months, even before we met formally, we were drawn to one another, tuning in to each other's presence across a cavernous lecture hall in a class of over two hundred students, though neither of us had any inkling of the other's attraction. For me, it was physical attraction; whereas she described intrigue with this long-haired hippie-like character who casually strolled in late, took a seat right in front of the professor, and matter-of-factly posed questions and interjected comments.

We were friends for two years before anything romantic evolved. She grew up the hard way, in a challenged and challenging family, and demonstrated a phenomenal resiliency, growing far beyond her upbringing. From the time I could remember, I was programmed to go to college. She had been actively discouraged from going to college. She did it almost entirely on her own, and after several starts and stops across five schools, she became the first person in her family to graduate from college.

She was not an addict, and never used like I did. She had a core of honesty and integrity that I marveled at, but could only aspire to. We had planned to move back East together prior to my arrest, and surprisingly she still came, leaving her own master's program in vocational counseling at Cal State San Francisco in the process. I absolutely adored her, and in the aftershock of my self-inflicted trauma, I would have been lost without her, and whether or not she was aware of that, she was extremely intuitive and likely sensed it. Knowing me in all the ways she did, joining me in New York was either an act of pure mercy or a desire to see some of the potential that she saw in me actualized, or some of both.

We got married during Labor Day weekend, and the following Tuesday I started as a diagnostic caseworker at St. Mary's Family and Children's Services, a residential treatment center in Syosset, NY, for latency-age and adolescent boys from all over Long Island and the five boroughs of New York City. I got the job in part because they saw me as a diamond in the rough that they could train, and in part because I was willing to accept the $12,500 annual salary—even in 1984, that was a near poverty-level wage.

I was part of a five-person multidisciplinary treatment team in a ninety-day diagnostic unit that conducted comprehensive evaluations and made placement recommendations on kids who were removed from their homes due to abuse, neglect, or juvenile delinquency. I performed psycho-social assessments, made home visits, and represented the agency in the family courts of the six counties from which our clients came. I saw some grotesque, stomach-churning examples of child abuse, the most heinous of which was a fourteen year-old whose fingers on both hands ended after the first knuckle. When he was six years old, his crack-addicted mother's crack-addicted boyfriend had held this child's hands over an open stove flame until, even after multiple surgeries, that was all that remained.

It quickly became clear that if I was going to continue in this area of work, I needed to get an advanced degree. I weighed the options of a master's in social work versus a doctorate in psychology, and based on bang for the bucks in terms of money and time, decided on an MSW at the Hunter College School of Social Work in Manhattan. I was also accepted to the prestigious MSW programs at Columbia University and NYU, but at that time the annual tuition was $9,600.00 at Columbia and $7,500.00 at NYU. Because the School of Social Work at Hunter was part of the City University of New York, tuition there was $1,900.00 annually. All three were among the most highly rated graduate schools of social work in the country, and the ratio of cost to quality made the Hunter program the most competitive of the three to get into.

I received my MSW in 1987, and was released from probation in May of 1988 with a Certificate of Relief from Disabilities, restoring all of the civil rights that were forfeited as a result of my felony conviction. I had stopped using intravenously. I snorted heroin and cocaine a small handful of times before forsaking them altogether in the late 1980s. But I continued to drink and smoke pot.

chapter five

[A PERSONAL PRISON IN]
PRIVATE PURGATORY

"A man who carries a cat by the tail learns
something he can learn in no other way."

MARK TWAIN

No one expects to become addicted to drugs (or anything else for that matter). Nobody ever plans to become an addict. Addiction is an insidious and patient disease. Although it overtakes some people with great speed, pinning them to the mat in a matter of a few short months or in some cases weeks, usually it bides its time. Addiction can pull people in slowly; its seduction so gradual that people often have no idea they're falling under its spell. In Greek mythology, the Sirens were fabled seductresses whose enchanting songs lured sailors on nearby ships to their deaths.

The sailors were so entranced that they never knew they were in danger until their vessels crashed against the rocky coast of the Sirens' island and sank. So it is with addiction; by the time most people have any clue that they're in trouble, they're already in too deep.

What began for me as an intermittent path to pleasure, as well as a transitory escape—initially from the stresses of life, and subsequently from emotional and physical pain—grew into a dogged preoccupation that over time metastasized into an obsession and a ruthless compulsion. I started out gently floating on a raft off a beach in the Caribbean and ended up being blown out to sea and lost in the middle of the ocean during a typhoon. My using began as a vacation and turned into a kidnapping, with a compelling case of Stockholm syndrome.

After completing my master's degree, I became credentialed as a Certified Social Worker in New York State (licensure was not yet an option) and went to work as a therapist at an outpatient psychiatric clinic for adolescents and young adults. The Youth Counseling League was located in a brownstone on 19th Street around the corner from Third Avenue in the Gramercy Park section of Manhattan. The approach to psychotherapy there was explicitly psychodynamic—an offshoot of psychoanalysis and psychoanalytic psychotherapy. The attention to supervision and training was phenomenal. The agency provided an intensive training program in psychodynamic theory and practice. It was like working at a postgraduate institute.

As rich as the learning environment was at the Youth Counseling League, the commute absolutely sucked. My wife and I lived in a basement apartment at my in-laws house in Fort Lee, New Jersey, so I would take the bus over the George Washington Bridge to 175th Street in upper Manhattan, where I would get on the subway and take the A train down to 14th Street, transfer to the L train and take that to Union Square, from which I would walk the handful of blocks east. After work, I would reverse the same route. It took about ninety minutes each way, and that was when the mass transit system functioned well. When it didn't, the trip could, and often did, take two hours or longer.

Our first daughter was born in the fall of 1987, shortly after I started at the Youth Counseling League. Watching her enter the world, I knew that my life and my priorities would never be the same. I was twenty-eight years old and felt nowhere near ready for my new role as a parent with its profound responsibilities. I came into it with an awareness of the downside—the challenges as far as how much time and difficulty parenting would likely involve. What I had absolutely no sense of, until I experienced it directly, was the breadth and depth of the rewards I would receive in trade. The connection I felt upon meeting my daughter transcends my ability to describe it. I experienced a love beyond anything I had ever known.

I gravitated toward employment closer to home and closer to an area of work with which I was intimately familiar, though not yet from a professional perspective: substance abuse. Less than two years removed from my master's program, twists of fate put me in the clinical director's position at Network, a residential substance abuse treatment program for adolescents in Rockleigh, NJ, a scenic twenty minute commute by car. There was no way in hell I felt ready for such a huge step up the career ladder, but the executive director strongly believed in me and, as brief as it was, my prior training and experience had prepared me well. The 25 percent jump in salary wasn't exactly a disincentive either.

The program had access to a gymnasium with a basketball court for client recreation. Although specific staff was assigned to supervise recreational activities, I made it a point to play hoops with the clients when my schedule allowed. I dubbed this treatment method "court counseling." It was a decidedly nontraditional though effective way to establish and deepen relationships with clients, particularly those who were standoffish and difficult to reach.

That a mainstream-appearing and height-challenged authority figure would get out from behind the big desk, exchange the jacket and tie for t-shirt and gym shorts, and rock 'n' roll with them made a compelling impression and engendered considerable respect. It didn't hurt that I was in my early thirties and still had some serious game. I found that I could develop more therapeutic rapport in half-an-hour on the basketball court than in two weeks of interactions in the regular treatment setting. This proved to be an important investment that paid dividends whenever those clients acted out in ways that required administrative intervention.

I could also talk with clients about the acute aftereffects of the full range of drugs with the type of gravitas and fluent detail that can only be birthed by direct personal experience. As is typical of clients in treatment for substance abuse, they wanted to know if I was in recovery myself.

My clinical training had oriented me to the pitfalls of answering such questions directly and schooled me in the tactical art of answering questions with questions. This technique serves several therapeutically useful purposes: it's an indirect means to gather additional information from clients; it deflects clients' attempts to take the immediate focus off of their issues; and, eventually realizing that they are not going to get a direct answer, they become frustrated and drop the subject. It had the secondary gain of enabling me to avoid answering a question that invariably made me uncomfortable because it was too damn close to home.

In addition to accumulating experience in substance abuse treatment, I sought out continuing education at every opportunity—workshops, conferences, seminars. Through a combination of experience, education, and passing written and oral exams, I attained my first state certification in substance abuse counseling in 1990.

We bought our first home in the little village of West Haverstraw close to the Hudson River in Rockland County, NY, and in 1992, I became the clinical director of the Chemical Dependency Unit (CDU) at Good

Samaritan Hospital Medical Center in Suffern, NY. CDU provided medically supervised detoxification and inpatient treatment for adults. I worked closely with the program director, the director of nursing, and the medical director, as well as supervised the entire clinical staff of counselors and social workers who conducted the individual, group, and family therapy.

Even though this program was located thirty-five miles northwest of New York City, due in part to our reputation and in part to the existing turf-focused politics of New York State licensure for "substance abuse" versus "alcoholism" treatment facilities, the majority of our referrals came from the most socioeconomically challenged communities in the city's five boroughs. We treated a great many men and women of color who came from neighborhoods that resembled war zones, ravaged by poverty, violence, and the multigenerational transmission of addiction.

A staggering number of our patients had experienced multiple, complex traumas. Too many had been victims of violent crime and quite a few had perpetrated acts of serious violence themselves. Not surprisingly, most of the perpetrators had previously been victims. It was not unusual for our patients to have served significant time in prison, with the threat of a return trip hanging over their heads. Many of them were HIV-positive, at a time when that disease was nowhere near as well understood as it is today.

A couple of months after I started "Good Sam," our younger daughter was born. My wife's labor during our first daughter's birth had been long and arduous, so in preparation for our next child I did childbirth-focused hypnosis and guided imagery with her. When she went into labor, she was able to draw on this preparation and use it as a resource. As a rule, second births tend to be easier and have shorter labors, but we were both amazed when our second daughter came into the world a mere five hours later, accompanied by much less pain.

Subsequently, I completed advanced training in clinical hypnotherapy and became nationally certified in that discipline. In consultation with the hospital's chief of anesthesiology, I began to do hypnotherapy with patients suffering with acute and chronic pain through the hospital's outpatient mental health clinic. He had reached the limits of what he could do to treat the pain of these patients through conventional medicine and was open-minded and progressive enough to refer them to me to see if clinical hypnosis could help. The results were consistently positive enough to please the patients, impress the chief of anesthesiology, and surprise me.

Although I didn't use during the day, as soon as I returned home from work, like clockwork, I smoked a couple of big bong hits or half a joint and drank a beer (or two) or had a glass (or two) of red wine. During the day, I helped people struggling with addiction learn how to stop using and get into recovery, and at night, I fed my own addiction. On most weekends I started using by late morning/early afternoon and continued throughout the rest of the day and evening so as to maintain a consistent "therapeutic" blood level.

From time to time the inevitable cognitive dissonance preyed on me, and deep down I felt like a hypocrite, but I continued to suppress it. During this period, I convinced myself that I smoked pot and drank in this manner because I wanted to, but the reality was that I needed to. Addiction is a function of the relationship between a person and the object(s) of his or her addiction, and I had an obsessive-compulsive relationship with pot and alcohol. I used every day, and whenever I didn't have what I needed, irritability, anxiety, upset, and pangs of withdrawal quickly ensued.

While we had both grown up in the New York metropolitan area and our families remained there, my wife and I maintained a desire to move back out West, where the pace of life is a little slower and the sun shines a whole hell of a lot more. When I was at Good Samaritan Hospital, my wife worked for Columbia University. We relocated to Tucson in 1997, when she was offered a position at the Biosphere after Columbia took over the management of that facility, hoping to turn it into a world-class research and educational center. A few months later, I was the director of clinical services (a title that would morph into vice president of counseling services when the agency's senior management structure changed) at Jewish Family & Children's Service of Southern Arizona.

In the fall of 1998, I started to have severe sciatic nerve pain shooting from my lower back all the way down my right leg. Initially, I saw this as no big deal since I had experienced a handful of similar bouts of sciatica over the previous twenty or so years. Each time it lasted anywhere from a few days to a couple of weeks before disappearing as suddenly as it had made its appearance. This time was different. Five weeks after the pain began, the cringe-inducing electrical current was still running the length of my leg with the same intensity.

An MRI revealed a herniated disc in my lumbar spine at the L-5 vertebrae and another disc protruding just below it at S-1. While the cause would remain uncertain, circumstantial evidence pointed toward the cumulative effects of a lifetime's worth of sports-related injuries, stresses, and strains, as well as twelve residential moves over the course of the preceding twenty years that had me carrying furniture that was too heavy while not paying enough attention to sound body mechanics. Within a week, I found myself in the office of a physician who specialized in pain management discussing treatment options.

We agreed that my treatment would include physical therapy and lumbar steroid injections as needed, but its underpinning would be a substantial ongoing prescription of opioids, to be reauthorized each month by the doctor. I vividly remember hearing him say the drug and dose he was starting me with, and immediately being of two dramatically different minds—one was ecstatic, the other full of trepidation—foremost was, *Yeah baby; bring it on!* Followed closely by, *Uh oh, this could be serious trouble.*

My ambivalence had nothing to do with my technical knowledge of the addictive potential of opioids, and everything to do with a cognizance of my ineluctable attraction to them. The realization that the ongoing availability of narcotics could unleash the most destructive features of a monster I wanted to believe I had successfully sidelined, was staring me dead in the face. Feeling the fear making a fist in my gut, I swallowed hard. Part of me knew way too well that this had the potential to be disastrous and that going down this road was really a fucking bad idea. Awareness like this only reveals itself to those who have a propensity for, if not a demonstrated history of, addiction. Of course, I squashed it.

My chronic pain gave me medical sanction—a license—to use my dope of preference. Owing to an amalgam of genuine pain, the physiological tolerance that opioids produce, and my desire for *more*, my prescriptions escalated in quantity, dosage, and psychoactive ingredients, progressing from hydrocodone (Vicodin) to oxycodone (Percocet), to a combination of oxycodone and fentanyl. Oxycodone is approximately one-and-a-half times the strength of hydrocodone. Fentanyl is a weapons-grade synthetic narcotic; comparable to heroin in potency, it's the strongest prescription painkiller available. It's so strong that dosages are measured in micrograms—one-millionth of a gram, instead of the usual milligrams—one-thousands of a gram. Generally used to treat patients with especially severe pain or for postsurgical pain management, it is sometimes used to treat people with chronic pain who are physically tolerant to opiates.

The fentanyl was prescribed in long-acting form—a transdermal patch that works by releasing the drug through the skin into body fats, which then slowly release it into the bloodstream over the course of seventy-two hours. The oxycodone was prescribed in its conventional short-acting pill form to supplement the fentanyl, just in case I had "breakthrough" pain. As far as I was concerned, there was always going to be enough breakthrough pain to justify the additional opioids.

The medical advantage of transdermal delivery over other routes of administration such as oral, topical, intravenous, intramuscular, etc. is that it is designed to provide a consistent controlled release of the drug. I wore the fentanyl patch as prescribed for the first two months. I figured that with timed-release fentanyl leeching into my bloodstream as a backstop, I could "play" with the oxycodone, taking it as I damn well pleased without having to worry about the horrors of withdrawal when I exhausted a month's supply of pills in sixteen to twenty-five or so days.

It seemed like a brilliant plan, the best of all worlds. But active addiction is a monstrosity with an appetite for *more* that is never sated longer than momentarily. Consequently, addicts can be incredibly resourceful, and one of our areas of expertise is finding ways to potentiate the acute effects of drugs. We will invariably find the most direct route to the target site of the brain to expedite the speed and maximize the effect of the drug's mechanism of action.

When it comes to substance use and its mood-altering impact, nonaddicts are content to hit singles, whereas those of us who have crossed the threshold into addiction swing for the fences. Mere base hits leave us wanting. If absolutely necessary we'll accept them, but we are determined to hit home runs, knocking the ball out of the park whenever possible.

It occurred to me that I could circumvent the fentanyl patch's timed-release mechanism and direct this elixir of euphoria into my bloodstream and my brain with much greater speed and intensity. Once again, part of me knew this was a bad idea that could go horribly wrong. And one more time, it didn't make a damn bit of difference. The controlled release element was easy to defeat.

Addiction begins with the mood-changing effects of substances. At first, people often experience positive effects by using drugs to change the way they feel. Through using they feel "good" or "better." Many drugs of abuse produce distinct feelings of pleasure, some of which are especially striking and powerful. Using helps people temporarily avoid or lessen mental, emotional, and physical distress. Drugs provide a way to turn down the volume of uncomfortable, painful sensations such as anxiety, fear, depression, physical pain, anger, boredom, loneliness, and stress.

However, when this way of temporarily easing, numbing, or blocking out discomfort turns into an ongoing way to cope with life's challenges and becomes a primary coping strategy, using is no longer voluntary.

The word *addiction* originated in ancient Rome. In Roman law, addiction was a formal award of a person or thing to another person—effectively a surrender to a master. Slaves given to Roman soldiers to reward them for performance in battle were known as addicts. Over time this definition was generalized so that a person who was viewed as a slave to anything became known as an addict.

Initially, the decision to use is a conscious choice, but as addiction progressively takes over a person's life, he or she loses more and more of the ability to exercise control over his or her thoughts, feelings, impulses, and actions. The ability to make conscious choices fades as the unconscious influences of the reward system located deep within the primitive survival-focused midbrain overrides the sophisticated decision-making abilities of the more highly evolved prefrontal cortex. At a certain point in the progression of active addiction, beneath the surface of conscious awareness, drug taking becomes equated with survival. The need to use assumes highest priority, becoming so strong that it suffocates all other needs. What originated as an experience that provides temporary freedom from the stresses and hassles of everyday life has evolved into a prison.

Addiction is a brain disease. It is considered a disorder of the brain because addiction actually changes the brain's structure and functioning. The National Institute on Drug Abuse (NIDA) of the US Department of Health and Human Services defines addiction as a "chronic, relapsing brain disease characterized by compulsive drug seeking and use, despite harmful consequences."

In 2011, the American Society of Addiction Medicine (ASAM) revised its definition of addiction, classifying it as a primary chronic disease of the brain's circuitry related to reward, motivation, and memory, rather than simply a problem based in behavior. This brain dysfunction is reflected in impaired behavioral control, craving for the object(s) of addiction, and the inability to abstain consistently, as well as diminished recognition of significant problems with one's behaviors and interpersonal relationships.

The use of drugs and mood-altering behaviors directly affects the brain by changing how it sends and receives information. The brain uses a communication system that sends and receives messages through certain naturally occurring chemicals known as neurotransmitters. When the "reward system," located deep within a part of the brain called the limbic system, is activated through messages sent by particular neurotransmitters, people experience pleasure. It is this stimulation of the brain's reward system that produces the mood-changing effects sought by people through drugs and behaviors. Research has been very clear that drug use effectively carjacks the brain's reward system by changing the levels of specific neurotransmitters—think of the reward system on steroids.

Brain imaging studies provide empirical evidence that addicts experience physical changes in the areas of their brains that involve judgment, decision-making, learning and memory, and behavior control. These changes affect how the brain works in extremely important ways. They help to explain the cycle of obsessive thinking, compulsive actions, and self-centered inability to delay gratification (including the decreased capacity to consider the consequences of one's actions) in which addiction traps those who struggle with it.

Opioid pain medications belong to the same class of substances as heroin (developed by the Bayer Company in Germany during the late 1890s as both a cough remedy and painkiller—comically, it was initially touted as a nonaddictive alternative to morphine). Like all drugs derived naturally or synthetically from the chemistry of the opium poppy, the two most prominent effects of these medications are pain relief and enhanced mood.

The analgesic effects of opioids are due to decreased perception of pain, reduced reaction to pain, and increased pain tolerance. Opioids work by binding to the brain's opiate receptors, which just happen to be highly concentrated in the areas that regulate pain and emotions. The activation of opiate receptors increases the level of dopamine in the brain, producing a state of euphoria and relaxation, along with the experience of pain diminution.

Dopamine is a neurotransmitter that plays a central role in the brain's reward system, affecting the processes related to the experience of pleasure and pain, the regulation of emotions, and physical movement. The use of opioids is complicated by this unusual coupling of relief and reward: relief from physical pain combined with the reward of euphoria and mood enhancement—both of which help to relieve emotional pain.

Within two to three months of beginning my opioid pain medication regime, I fell into a pattern of using my meds as a generalized chemical coping method. As a teenager I learned that I could change the way I felt by getting high, and as an adult, I knew my meds were a vehicle to effectively plan and control my feelings. Rather than be subjected to their distressing whims, I could dose myself to feel good or at least better.

Chronic pain evokes intense emotions. I was frustrated and angry that I was in pain so often. I was mired in self-pity and resentment as to why this happened to me. I was sad and depressed because physically I was unable to do some of the things that had been a regular and important part of my life. I was anxious and fearful about what activities would increase my pain and how my limitations would affect me in the future. I was wracked with guilt and remorse at my attenuated ability to be physically and emotionally available to my family, especially my kids.

Because physical pain was my legitimate pathway to using, it became my central feeling state. Emotional discomfort in any form fused with my physical pain. As a result of the intimacy of the mind-body connection, my emotional pain and physical pain exacerbated each other. I took my opioids in response to physical pain, but I also took them when I felt anxious, irritable, sad, frustrated, angry, fearful, depressed, stressed, etc. The meds took the rough edges off my emotions, as well as my pain, granting me a blessed temporary reprieve from them. I spent as much time in a state of comfortable numbness as I could. Shit, if I could have, I would have resided there permanently.

One of the shortcomings of mind- and mood-altering substances is that they always wear off. But the effects don't just subside, returning me to the baseline state I was in prior to seeking chemical refuge. One of the inexorable dynamics of dope in any form—whether from the street like crack, prescribed by a doctor like painkillers, or bought at a store like alcohol—is that the relief it provides is all-too-soon replaced by a worsening of the state one was in when the substance was ingested. My use of medically prescribed opioids became a vicious circle of cause and effect. I used to dull my physical and emotional pain, and the aftermath of using only created more emotional pain, driving me to use even more.

The brain adapts to repetitive experiences by forming memory connections or tracks that are unconscious. When such repetitive experiences revolve around using, the unconscious memory tracks that are laid are the neurological foundation of the "habits" of addiction. Such habits can be so difficult to control because they are created by changes in brain functioning and work in the brain's operating system—outside of conscious awareness. The intense cravings that addicts experience for their substance or activity of preference, sometimes long after they last used, are an example of the strength of these memory tracks.

The progression of active addiction is a lot like pushing a wheelbarrow in a rut. The more the wheelbarrow is pushed in the rut through time and repetition, the more well-established that rut becomes. The more well-established and deeper the rut becomes, the harder it is to get the wheelbarrow out. There comes a tipping point where it becomes much harder to get the wheelbarrow out of the rut than to continue to follow it, which only makes it deeper still.

Positive reinforcement—the desired outcome that results from using—for example, feeling "good" or "better," is one form of this process. Each time using results in the desired outcome, the memory tracks that link the object(s) of addiction with that result become stronger. Positive reinforcement teaches people to repeat the same behaviors in order to get the same results. The more the process is repeated, the greater the chances are that it will continue to be repeated.

Conditioning is another example of such neuroadaptation. Certain emotional states and situations, including specific people and places, become connected with the experience of using and can light the fire of obsessive thoughts, compulsive behaviors, and self-centered tunnel-vision linked to using. As a result, coming into contact with the emotional states or people and places associated with using increases the odds that someone will use.

The brain connects emotion, memory, and sensory stimuli, linking experiences perceived as "positive" with specific images, sounds, smells, and textures, coding them as omens of comfort and reward. These unconscious learned responses are strong enough that they remain operative even after years of abstinence. As a result, their memory tracks tend to pull people back toward the experiences and behaviors with which they are familiar and comfortable, making it more difficult to stop such behaviors and stay stopped. Like petroglyphs etched in rock formations that are clearly visible hundreds of years later, the rhapsodic recollections of early drug use are engraved deep within the midbrain—beckoning sweetly and seductively.

The opioids I took for my chronic pain poured gasoline on the slow burning embers of an active addiction that I had mollified for a decade and a half with daily use of marijuana and alcohol. I had watched the use of so-called hard drugs fade from sight in the rearview mirror of my past. The last time I had done cocaine was at my ten year high school reunion in late November of 1987. My wife let me fly solo while she stayed with my parents and took care of our newborn daughter. It was ridiculous how many people came to the reunion armed with piles of blow. It was an occasion of Dionysian excess. Snorting was the only route of administration that evening, and I had more than my fill until 6:30

the following morning when first one, then the other of my nostrils shut down, my body telling me in no uncertain terms that I was done.

Without knowing how depraved the festivities would be, but knowing in advance that I would have no business attempting to drive home afterward, my brother had generously offered to pick me up wherever I was and drive me back to our parents' house. As the sun rose higher, I staggered up the stairs to a spare bedroom and crash-landed on the bed. I labored to breathe through my mouth since my nose was unavailable. Acute cocaine withdrawal always made my skin crawl, and that nasty, physically exhausted, mentally wired, coming-down-from-coke-feeling was beating the shit out of me. Just then my wife walked in, placed our six-week-old daughter on my chest, and left the room without saying a word. No less clear than this passive-aggressive flourish was the awareness that the tectonic plates of my world had shifted irreversibly.

Those plates began to shift under my feet again as my use of the opioids prescribed for my chronic pain became increasingly beyond my control. Significant shifts in the tectonic plates that comprise the Earth's crust can cause earthquakes and volcanic activity. My obsessive preoccupation with and compulsive use of narcotics began to collide with my need to believe that my prior personal experiences and my professional knowledge inoculated me against such things. My addiction was really a volcano that, in spite of continuous low-level magma activity, had been in a period of relative dormancy. The eruption was now in progress.

I had essentially transitioned from using street drugs to socially acceptable, medically prescribed dope. It was just me, my prescribing physician, and the prescription-filling pharmacy. It was all medically sanctioned and perfectly legal. Yet it still took me to places—physically, mentally, emotionally, and spiritually—that were eerily reminiscent of shooting heroin daily during much of 1981–82.

Another piercing reminder of that era came in 2002 when the results of some annual blood work came up out of whack for my liver functions. My doctor ordered the tests repeated and the results were the same, leading to another test looking for specific genetic material. I was diagnosed with Hepatitis C, a delayed consequence of sharing needles with an eclectic cross-section of humanity, brought together for one purpose and one purpose only. In the face of this intimidating diagnosis, I found myself experiencing gratitude that it wasn't worse. Some of those I had used with intravenously had been infected with the HIV virus, gotten AIDS, and died.

chapter six

[NO MATTER WHERE YOU GO,] THERE YOU ARE

"You carry your pain wherever you go
Full of the blues, and trying to lose
You ain't going to learn what you don't want to know."
JOHN BARLOW, *BLACK-THROATED WIND*, GRATEFUL DEAD

Like constant companions, everywhere I went, my pain and my addiction went with me. During the winter of 2000, when I was Vice President of Counseling Services at Jewish Family & Children's Service of Southern Arizona, I was graced with the opportunity to travel to Israel with a group of other professionals from several different organizations in Tucson.

Being an avid student of news and current events, a behavioral health professional with kids, and a practicing addict, this trip necessitated some special preparations. At that time, the terrorist attacks and spasms of serious violence that rocked Israel during the first Palestinian Intifada of the mid-late 1990s had subsided. This notwithstanding, the potential for close encounters with terrorism or other forms violence was inherent in traveling to this part of the world, so I took the extraordinary step of making a video tape for my daughters, who were then thirteen and eight years old respectively.

It was a "good-bye" message, just in case, god forbid. I wanted to make certain that in the event anything happened to me and I didn't return, my daughters would hear and know directly from me that I loved them with all my heart, and that I was incredibly proud of them. My wife taped me as I spoke to the video camera. It was surreal, yet profoundly real, and deeply emotional as I found myself tearing up more than once.

Based on my usual opioid pain medication refill schedule, I was due to renew my prescription about halfway through the trip. Obviously, that was unacceptable and alternate arrangements had to be made. I carefully constructed a letter to my prescribing physician that accurately described this trip as an once-in-a-lifetime opportunity, the timing of which coincidentally happened to justify a substantial deviation in the timing of my next refill.

Given the intense physical rigors that go along with such an extraordinary trip, it was realistic to expect increased pain levels. Moreover, even taking my meds as prescribed (as if that would ever happen), I'd run out and begin the horror show of full-blown withdrawal somewhere between Jerusalem and the Sea of Galilee. My doctor agreed that giving me another full prescription a week early was an unavoidable necessity of circumstance. Little did he know that I had already run through my current prescription after just three weeks and needed the new script to avoid getting dope sick right then.

The trip was an astounding experience—twelve days of exploring the area where so many events involved in shaping the history of our world and three of its major religions took place. We traveled all over Israel, staying overnight in Jerusalem, Tel Aviv, and a kibbutz at the tip of northern Israel overlooking parts of Lebanon and Syria.

For most of this adventure, we had two excellent guides who treated our group to a wealth of information covering the cultural, ethnic, religious, political, and socioeconomic history, contemporary issues, and extraordinary challenges of the Holy Land. We visited the Sea of Galilee and the Golan Heights, as well as the West Bank, where we met at length with representatives of both the right-wing settler movement and the left-leaning Peace Now initiative.

I prayed at the Western Wall (a.k.a. the "Wailing" Wall)—the last remnant of Jerusalem's massive Jewish Temple complex, which was originally built by Solomon atop the Temple Mount in the tenth century BCE and destroyed by the Babylonians in 586 BCE. The Second Temple was dedicated on the same site in 516 BCE and expanded significantly to include the construction of the Western Wall by Herod around 19 BCE, before being destroyed by the Romans in 70 CE. Running my hands over its majestic rough hewn stone was like plugging into a USB port to 3,000 years of ancestral history.

At the Church of the Holy Sepulcher, built during the fourth century CE, I climbed the steps that millions of people over the course of centuries had climbed before me to touch the rock that is said to have held the cross on which Jesus was crucified. Even though the steps are solid rock they are noticeably worn in shapes that resemble footsteps due to the unrelenting parade of people making pilgrimage to this sacred place.

I went to the lowest place on Earth, literally, the Dead Sea, at 1,300 feet below sea level. It was an overcast, cold, and gloomy day. The weather was inhospitable enough that just three of our party dared to swim. Although ordinarily it was way too cold for me to contemplate swimming, there was nothing ordinary about this scenario. It was the fucking Dead Sea, and I had no idea if I'd ever be there again, so I was damn sure going in! One of the unique aspects of this particular body of water is that the salt content is so high (the main reason it's biologically "dead") that you don't sink in it. You can't help but naturally float, without any effort. I took advantage of this unusual experience by leaning back, crossing my legs, and reading parts of the Jerusalem English-language newspaper while I floated leisurely.

I was well aware of how blessed I was to be on such an excursion, and profoundly grateful for it. And yet, as remarkable as every day was, each one unfolding to reveal mind-blowing, once-in-a-lifetime experiences, there lurking in the shadows at nearly all times was the level of opioids coursing through my central nervous system, the status of my stash, and an obsessive preoccupation with my next dose.

As always, I had gone through the exercise of carefully crafting a dosing schedule to plan out how many meds I could take on a daily basis and how best to distribute them during the course of each day so that they would last the entire trip. Deviating from it almost immediately, I ran through meds that were prescribed to last a month in eight and a half days. Another fine plan blown to hell—my only priority was to make my opioids last through the trip and the first few days of what I anticipated to be massive jet lag at home. I figured I'd end up suffering through my usual shake-and-bake self-detox dance after that.

It took six more years before I would fully accept the reality that I was constitutionally incapable of taking opioids as prescribed. One of the reasons for this innate inability is that I suffered from a rare and very specific form of dyslexia—the only area of my life it affected was my ability to read certain prescriptions. Instead of "take one to two tablets every four to six hours," I invariably read, "take four to six tablets every one to two hours."

Having exhausted my own supply, I had three and a half days to negotiate somehow—detox during the trip needed to be avoided at all costs. Not only did I want to enjoy our final few days, but being in close company with influential professional colleagues, I needed to keep my act together.

Such situations necessitate the sort of resilient resourcefulness so familiar to many addicts. Somehow the ends always justify the means: the ends of having *enough* to catch a buzz, or at minimum to avoid getting dope sick, justify the means that usually involve some combination of deception and manipulation, everything from lying and stealing to manipulating through persuasion, pleading, or good old-fashioned bullshitting.

Active addicts have well-developed ways of assessing their environment, wherever they are, scanning for potential ways and means to use. Several days prior to running out of opioids, I had noticed, actually zeroed in on like an advanced radar tracking system, that the colleague with whom I was sharing a hotel room had a prescription for, wait for it—opioid painkillers. While I made an indelible mental note of this, my internal voice was comfortably encased in situation-specific denial, "Okay, they're there, but I won't need 'em. I have enough of my own." Yeah, right.

As if on autopilot, I immediately engaged in a familiar series of calculations focused on maximizing return relative to risk, along with a favorite rationalization to facilitate my action plan. Based on the prescription date and the number of pills remaining, he only used them sparingly and as absolutely necessary—how absurd. He obviously didn't *really* need them. As a result, he likely didn't track his inventory in any sort of careful or ongoing way. So, at the point at which I exhausted my own supply, I simply moved on to his, walking that tightrope of taking as many as I could without it being overtly noticeable.

That provided a decidedly lower dose that lasted for two days and kept me from being sick. For the final thirty-six hours of the trip I was reduced to playing up my pain due to the intensity of the trip (though this did have some validity—the most effective manipulations always do), and playing on the sympathy of a female colleague who had a script of Tylenol 3 with Codeine. I got her to give me most of what she had. They barely contained enough of the active ingredient I craved, but they kept the dope sickness at bay until I made it home to collapse in a haze of withdrawal and jet lag.

chapter seven

[YOU CAN'T SAVE YOUR FACE AND]
YOUR ASS AT THE SAME TIME

*"The truth you believe and cling to makes
you unavailable to hear anything new."*

PEMA CHÖDRÖN

We are destined to repeat the same experiences unless and until we learn the essential lessons they have to teach us. Once again, my life had devolved into the relentless pursuit of neurochemical reward and relief. Only now, I had much more to lose. Even with an amazing family—built on a marriage that represented a true partnership forged through rich and enduring love and one that had already survived some momentous challenges; two wonderful, well-adjusted, smart, and beautiful kids; and a thriving career—I fell into a grind of using in order to recreate the reward of the high, find relief from the pain, and avoid the dysphoria of the crash as the relief receded. More and more of my time, energy, and attention were consumed by my pain, thinking about using, using, recovering from the effects of using, and finding the ways and means to get and use more.

The planning of my day and all of my activities revolved around the availability of my opioids. And there were never enough. For me, when it came to the pain meds, there was no such thing as "enough." Each day I would commit to using a specific allotment of Percocet, and often by mid-day they were already gone. For the most part, as long as I produced the quality and quantity of work required of me, I could make my own work schedule. This flexibility gave me opportunities to return home to resupply. I lost count of the number of days when I left the house in the morning, determined to use no more than what I brought with me, only to find myself in my car heading home by lunch time to get more.

The lies, manipulations, and deceptions that I perpetrated as the ferocity of my addiction grew progressively eroded my wife's ability to trust me. She had the ability to read me like a children's book and could invariably tell when I was being less than honest. Every time I was dishonest with her—whether it was about how many meds I had used that day, why I needed to take extra meds today, or how many I had left for the month, etc.—it hurt her and hurt us. It was as if I was spilling drops of sulfuric acid on the foundation of our marriage. Intermittently, we would have moments when I would break down and commit to changing and to being a better person, to being the person she deserved me to be. I so wanted to be better—for her and for my daughters, and for periods of time I could pull it together. But it never lasted. The gravitational pull of that black hole would suck me back in.

I started keeping a good-sized chunk of the fentanyl patch in my mouth as a matter of course, giving me a much more direct and substantial dose. I would run clinical staff meetings and conduct individual supervision, as well as attend senior management meetings with my executive director/

CEO, chewing on a big-ass piece of fentanyl patch. Every so often it would get stuck in the back of my throat at an inopportune time and I'd have to dislodge it by maintaining the illusion that I was simply clearing my throat or coughing.

To accommodate my using, my sleeping pattern became bizarrely distorted. I usually woke up early to begin with—around 5:30 a.m., taking my time to leisurely sit and sip my coffee, watch some news, and meditate in preparation for the day ahead. I had been meditating daily for a number years, and continued this practice even as my active addiction escalated. As my using progressed, I started to get up at 3:30–4:00 a.m. so I could dose myself at the earliest possible opportunity, washing the day's inaugural Percocets down with my first cup of coffee, thus dissolving the pills faster and expediting the speed at which their effects washed over me.

I usually administered the last dose of the day as soon as I returned home from work. I had to go to bed absurdly early in order to get up at that ungodly hour so I could commence the new day of using with that all-important initial dose. I started to go to bed at 8:00 p.m., sometimes even 7:30 p.m. I attributed this to my pain, that I needed to lie down, etc., and sometimes it was, but more often it was really about using. I could see the confusion and concern in the expressions of my two daughters (then in their mid-teens and pre-adolescence respectively). Why was their father regularly going to bed long before they were?

As incomprehensible as it may sound, this state of affairs became completely normal to me. It's possible for just about any circumstance to become "normal," no matter how strange, different, or unhealthy it might seem. All it requires is enough exposure to get used to it. Through experience virtually anything can become familiar to the point where it seems normal. When I was twelve, my family spent a week during the summer with my maternal grandparents in the tiny town where they lived for many years in the southeast corner of Pennsylvania, close to the borders of both Delaware and Maryland. It was a bucolic setting with miles of rolling green hills and corn fields, an archetype of Mid-Atlantic farm country.

One day we visited a childhood friend of my mother's and her family on their 150-acre farm. As we drove up to the farm with the windows of our Chevy station wagon rolled down, I remember the first remnants of that smell wafting into the car and the alternating gagging and howling it elicited from my younger siblings and I. It was ghastly—an olfactory assault with what smelled like a deadly weapon that made it hard to breathe. When we were greeted as instant friends by the kids who lived there, the very first thing I said after "Hi" was "How do you stand the smell!" A boy who was about my age looked at me quizzically and replied, "What smell?"

Maintaining active addiction necessitates a set of defensive maneuvers to evade the natural corrective consequences of cognitive, behavioral, and ethical dissonance as the disease progresses. Addiction is especially insidious in how it convinces those of us who suffer from it that we do not have it. Those who become addicted almost always believe they can control their using, even in the face of blatant evidence to the contrary.

Defense mechanisms are psychological processes that operate unconsciously to help us cope with aspects of reality that are too painful or threatening to acknowledge. They are normal and universal features of the human mind that protect us from the awareness of thoughts, feelings, and facts that are uncomfortable or painful. Defense mechanisms provide shelter from the storm of distressing situations with which we cannot cope.

The use of defense mechanisms is natural and adaptive, and everyone uses them throughout life. Some means of protection from painful thoughts and experiences is important in order to remain mentally and emotionally healthy and functional—too much psychological pain is unhealthy, plain and simple. Defense mechanisms become unhealthy when their use causes problems. They can become overused, effectively overprotecting us from reality to the point where we become disconnected from it. When this happens, our defenses can enable all sorts of self-defeating and destructive behaviors, addiction being a prime example.

It is part of human nature to avoid painful truths, and it is part of the nature of active addiction that painful truths abound. Sometimes these truths lurk just beneath the surface of awareness. We may have a sense or know on some level that "something" is wrong, perhaps terribly wrong, but it is too damn painful to concede consciously.

These truths are kept at bay through a combination of the defenses of denial, minimizing, rationalizing, and avoidance. These phenomena help to protect addicts from mental and emotional pain related to their addiction and provide fuel for continuing to use even as the negative consequences continue to mount. In keeping addicts from being able to accurately see many of the problems that are obvious to others, these defense mechanisms create cognitive distortions and blind spots, similar to that space in a driver's field of vision somewhere between what's visible in either the rearview or the side view mirror. Often, it's what we can't see that poses the greatest danger.

Denial is perhaps the most well-known and common defense mechanism. It is an unconscious rejection of unacceptable feelings, needs, thoughts, or external reality factors. A situation that threatens emotional safety or sense of self is simply not perceived. People in denial seem to ignore distressing facts and discard information that contradicts what they need to believe, like an addict in active addiction who refuses to admit that he or she has a problem because this reality creates too much anxiety, stress, or pain. Denial keeps people from accurately seeing the full impact of their actions on their lives—it is too uncomfortable, too painful for them to admit to and accept.

As I described earlier, for many years during my active addiction, my denial manifested in a genuine belief that I was not an addict—despite ample evidence that I was. One of the most damaging effects of denial is how it impairs the capacity to appreciate the suffering active addiction causes others. I couldn't allow myself to believe that I was an addict, much less that my addiction was damaging my marriage and, despite rendering me less emotionally and physically available, harming my relationship with my kids. Moreover, I was unable to consider that my using impaired my professional performance.

Denial is often confused with dishonesty and the labyrinth of lies that active addiction ordinarily spawns, but the unconscious process of denial and overt dishonesty are two very different things. With conscious, deliberate dishonesty the individual remains aware of the difference between his or her own claims and the actual truth of the matter. Someone in denial, on the other hand, genuinely believes his or her own deceptions and distortions, and accordingly regards the divergent opinions of others as false, viewing their efforts to convince him or her otherwise as misguided at best and malicious at worst.

"You're a drug addict, and you need to do something about it."

"I'm not a drug addict, I'm responsible for over thirty behavioral health and substance abuse treatment programs and twenty therapists. I help drug addicts."

Minimizing is a scaled down (sort of a minor league) form of denial. Instead of negating the existence of a painful reality altogether, minimizing is an unconscious decreasing or lessening of the severity of such a situation/ event. It makes painful thoughts, emotions, behaviors, and situations more comfortable/less threatening than they really are. It's extremely common for addicts to minimize or under report how much they use, how often they use, and even what substances they use—I sure as hell did.

Rationalization is the effort to justify behaviors, feelings, thoughts, or desires that are unacceptable, thereby creating false but credible justifications. When one's actual motivations are not socially or publicly acceptable, rationalization operates by substituting more appropriate motives. For example, an addict admits to using daily, but only because his or her partner is nagging him or her, or that he or she is in pain, or that he or she is under great stress at work. My most frequent rationalizations involved the last two of these. In addition to being in continuous pain, the enormity of my job responsibilities created a ton of stress. This line of thought was unintentionally encouraged by one of my doctors who wrote in an assessment that without the aid of opioid pain meds, I might not be able to work full-time. That's what I'm talking about!

Avoidance is the unwillingness to encounter situations, people, or activities because they create anxiety, stress, or pain. It may also involve finding ways not to discuss or even think about distressing topics. Usually, it takes the form of removing oneself physically from a situation—such as not going home to face an angry partner, staying home from work to elude the boss, or avoiding places where someone to whom money is owed is likely to be.

In my case, there were times when I evaded my wife out of fear that she would be able to tell how loaded I was. I would also avoid situations and activities where my chronic pain was likely to bring me face-to-face with my physical limitations, as well as put them on display for others. Whereas I had always sought out opportunities to participate in anything sports-related, since I was physically unable to perform, or at least to perform to my satisfaction, I'd opt to just stay away.

Personally, my favorite defense mechanism has always been intellectualization—the unconscious controlling of emotions or impulses through excessive thinking about them rather than actually experiencing them. It uses logic and intellect to remain dispassionate, and consists of treating an emotionally charged situation in a detached or emotionally tamped-down way. The fact that I ran through a month's worth of pain meds in three weeks sucked because I had to self-detox one more time, but it was a situation to be problem-solved through more careful and well thought out planning. As my active addiction became increasingly beyond my control and my defensive fortifications were disintegrating, I kept trying to restrain the encroaching feelings of anxiety and fear by thinking I had enough intelligence and professional knowledge to keep the conflicting facets of my life together—even as they were clearly falling apart.

In July of 2004, I represented my agency at a four-day statewide conference on substance abuse in Sedona, Arizona. I had run out of meds on day one of this conference, and on day three I was in full-blown withdrawal while attending an afternoon workshop on buprenorphine. Buprenorphine is a semisynthetic opiate (actually a partial opioid agonist) approved by the FDA in 2002 for detoxification and opioid maintenance/ replacement therapy. It provides an alternative to methadone that has some significant advantages, including fewer side effects and lower addictive potential.

Opioid withdrawal syndrome varies in intensity with the level and duration of use. By this time, I had been using medically prescribed opioids daily for six years. The first signs of withdrawal occur shortly before the next *scheduled* dose—as if I ever waited until then. The peak of withdrawal occurs thirty-six to seventy-two hours after the last dose, and I was right around the forty-eight hour mark. As the presenter described the symptoms of opiate/opioid withdrawal one by one, I found myself experiencing them literally—in all of their excruciating detail: rhinorrhea (runny nose), lacrimation (watery eyes), muscle aches and spasms, sweating, chills, gooseflesh, stomach cramps, drug craving and obsession, restlessness, anxiety, and irritability. It was a grotesque tragicomedy, the irony as thick as the mucous saturating my nonstop runny nose.

There were never enough pain meds. No matter how many there were, there was no such thing as *enough*. The more I had, the more I took. Each month I ran out like clockwork, throwing myself into withdrawal. Opioid withdrawal felt like someone had taken an electric sander to every nerve ending in my body.

Since I went through it nearly every single goddamn month, I developed a well-practiced self-detox protocol. I had a prescription for the sleep medication Ambien, but as long as I had opioids, I slept just fine. I got the Ambien specifically for those days between when I ran out of pain meds and when I was able to have them refilled. Supplemented with copious quantities of pot and alcohol, the Ambien helped to turn down the volume of the screaming in my central nervous system. Even still, I was wretched.

Of course, the only thing that provided any real relief was more opioids. As Schedule II Controlled Substances, my prescriptions required reauthorization monthly. I'd always try to get my refills in advance of the thirty days the meds were supposed to last, straining to determine precisely how early I could request refills without arousing questions or concerns.

Periodically, I went to greater lengths to get more. As long as I can remember, my mother has had a prescription for opioids. A case of polio as a child that was mild enough to go undiagnosed nonetheless resulted in a slight curvature of her spine, which left her in chronic pain. She has been taking pain meds forever, and has to have a degree of physical dependence on them. However, she has never used them like I used them.

Because she took them as prescribed or less frequently, my mother regularly had opioids left over at the end of the month. During the early to mid-2000s, there were quite a few months when, after running out of my own meds, I beseeched her to send me whatever pain medication she could spare. I played the pain card, half-asking/half-pleading, drawing on my mother's sympathy and empathy. The next day, like clockwork I'd receive an express mail package, and I could breathe again . . . for the moment.

After so many of these phone calls (to say nothing of my prolific pilfering of her pills previously), she likely had at least some inkling that I had a problem. However, the family members and significant others of addicts also experience denial, minimization, rationalization, avoidance, and intellectualization. Having a child with a drug addiction is a painful truth few parents wish to acknowledge.

Sometimes she sent enough meds to easily last until I was due for a refill, and I thought to myself, I'll have enough. And almost always, I was wrong because there was a direct correlation—the more I had, the more I took. In this context, "enough" was a fast-moving target.

There was never enough because there is always a need for more. The need for more was my constant companion. In early December of 2004, it travelled with me to Phoenix for the Ninth International Congress on Ericksonian Approaches to Hypnosis and Psychotherapy. This is a renowned international conference held every few years since 1980, and I was surrounded by many of the biggest names and most influential theorists, practitioners, and authors in psychotherapy on the planet. While staying at the Hyatt Regency in downtown Phoenix, I ran out of meds and placed one of my disconsolate calls to my mother. The following day I picked up my express mail delivery at the concierge desk.

Over the course of my eight years running the behavioral health operations at JFCS, the number of clinical staff and programs grew by approximately 40 percent. During my tenure the annual budget for the Counseling Services department nearly tripled. I authored or coauthored grant proposals that were awarded over $3 million in funding. I designed and implemented a comprehensive system for measuring and evaluating client and program outcomes. And during this same time, my life came apart piece by piece.

In professional addiction assessment circles it is common knowledge that as a person's addiction worsens, the resulting adverse consequences affect life domains in a cascading sequence. It is a sequence I knew well, having taught it in clinical supervision and training: active addiction affects relationships with family and significant others first; health problems usually come next; and the last major life area to be seriously impacted tends to be job/career.

In my increasing desperation to stay medicated, I went places and crossed lines I never, ever would have believed possible. Each trespass was another step toward personal and professional self-destruction.

Somewhere inside I knew this, and kept going. There were times when the therapists in the Counseling Services Department (all of whom were under my clinical-administrative stewardship) would see me in obvious pain. Wanting to be of help, separately two such staff offered me unused painkillers. I knew damn well that taking their meds was a bright red line, the crossing of which represented an appalling violation of professional ethics, as well as the standards governing my state credentials in both social work and substance abuse counseling.

My internal self-talk lit up with air-horn volume warning signals. I knew this was a really fucking bad idea; that going "there" had way too much potential to bite me in the ass, putting everything that I had worked so hard and so long for in jeopardy. But I took them up on their offers anyway. I compounded this grievous mistake by going back to each of them on an additional occasion to get more. It was a betrayal of my profession, my agency, my CEO, my staff, my wife, and my children. The corrosion of my character was complete. I was buffeted by guilt and shame, but it was the fear of being found out and of the possible consequences that was most toxic. I soldiered on, relying on my disintegrating defense mechanisms to shield me from the swell of my own intrusive thoughts.

I was undone when one of the therapists from whom I received meds shared our "secret" with another member of the Counseling Services Department who was disgruntled, and on her way out the door to a new job disclosed to one of my fellow senior management team members what she had been told. The information made its way to the CEO, who had always been extremely supportive of me. Though clearly saddened and disappointed, she let me know matter-of-factly that this incident required reporting to the Arizona Board of Behavioral Health Examiners (AZBBHE).

I was sick at the idea of having to share what I had wrought with my wife. After carefully walking on the tightrope between behavioral health professional and practicing addict for so long, I completely lost my balance and was in free fall.

One would think that this was the appropriate time to admit to the drug addiction that I had kept shrouded in shadows. After all this time I had been presented with a clear opening to finally cop to it and get help. This was precisely what my wife had begged me to do for so many years. What the hell was there left to hide? What was left to hold on to? But no! I still wasn't ready to admit that I was an addict. I had neither the courage nor the humility to accept defeat. I was in such a deep hole, the only option I was capable of pursuing was to keep digging. I could feel my wife's heartsickness at my head-up-my-ass unwillingness to acquiesce to the obvious, and sensed that this was a further tipping point in our marriage, pushing it closer to the edge—yet I remained stuck in this dead end of my own creation.

The position I took with the AZBBHE was that I wasn't an addict, but rather someone whose chronic pain wasn't always well managed, and that my pain had led me to exercise poor judgment and decision-making in these few specific, unfortunate instances. How's that for intellectualization? I stopped smoking pot immediately after being reported to the board. At the time I was forty-four and had smoked pot since the age of twelve, and virtually every day since I was sixteen (literally missing only a handful of days here and there). This was a really big deal for me, but I knew I'd have to undergo urinalysis and while all other drugs left the body after about seventy-two hours, reefer metabolizes into the fatty tissue and can be detected for at least thirty days after last use. Testing positive for pot would surely interfere with my argument that I wasn't an addict.

Going before the state board was devastating. Such regulatory entities exist to protect public safety, to ensure standards of professional education, training, and ethical conduct. These are necessary and important functions. I had made grievous mistakes and expected to be hammered for them, but what I experienced was a demonization for which I was wholly unprepared.

The board staff suggested it was unnecessary to have an attorney to represent my interests at the initial face-to-face meeting that it had labeled "informal." Within minutes, as the tone became increasingly castigating and the atmosphere grew explicitly punitive, it became apparent that not having an attorney was a serious error and that I needed one ASAP. I was treated as if I had had sex with a client. I was traumatized, and with each in-person contact I had with the board, I was re-traumatized. At one point, the attorney I retained, who had extensive experience with this board, told me directly that he had never seen the then Executive Director go after someone as personally as she seemed to in my case. There was no fact-based explanation for this. It was as though I reminded her of an ex-husband or boyfriend who had done her wrong. I perceived myself to be a victim, but the bottom line was that I was a volunteer. And I was traumatized by the consequences of my own actions.

My situation was legitimately confounded by my chronic pain. I was genuinely worried about what would happen in the event I couldn't take opioid painkillers if I had to go to treatment. I had already presented the board with a formal substance abuse evaluation by a physician who was one of the Southwest's foremost experts in pain management and addiction. I had seen her every six months for the past couple of years as part of my overall pain treatment regime. The board required me to get an additional evaluation by a provider from their approved list. I paid nearly $1,000.00 out of pocket for a comprehensive substance abuse evaluation by the then head of the Arizona State Department of Health Services, who was also an addictionologist.

Being an experienced professional with the ability to speak the same language enabled me to manipulate the doctors conducting these evaluations. Both came to the conclusions I wanted—that I suffered from a chronic pain condition that wasn't always well-managed, and as a result my pain led me to exercise poor judgment and decision-making. But I was not an addict. In spite of being so out of control, I was still trying desperately to hang on to my opioids and to control the outcome.

This would prove to be an excellent example of the need to be careful what you wish for. I won this battle en route to losing the war. My social work license was placed on probation for a minimum of one year, during which I was mandated to complete a graduate-level ethics class; attend weekly psychotherapy with progress reports submitted to the board monthly; and call a 1-800 number every morning—if the number on the recorded message matched the last digit of my social security number, I had to report to an approved site for random piss-testing by 1:00 p.m. that day.

Consistent with the results of my substance abuse evaluations, my probation agreement with the AZBBHE allowed me to continue to use my prescribed opioids. Although my professional license was on a carefully monitored probation regime, I still had medical and regulatory sanction to use my dope of choice. In fact, I could potentially find myself in deeper shit if, on urinalysis, I *didn't* come up positive for oxycodone (the psychoactive ingredient in Percocet) and fentanyl.

As described earlier, defense mechanisms protect us from too much pain. For everyone, but for addicts in particular, the painful realities our defenses safeguard us from include threats to our self-image, known in certain circles as "face." I had to learn the hard way the wisdom of the twelve-step saying: "You can't save your face and your ass at the same time."

The concept of "face" is Asian in origin. In English, face equates to reputation, status, prestige, and honor. It is the positive social value a person can effectively claim for him- or herself—the respectability a person is given by others, based on variables such as what they do (employment/career), what they have (socioeconomic status/material possessions), and who they are (family of origin, family of procreation, and personal conduct).

Face is something in which many people are emotionally invested. Far from static, it is a dynamic entity that evolves over time, and can be maintained, enhanced, diminished, or lost depending upon events and interactions. Face was a sense of worth that came in large part from my professional life, reflecting my ongoing concerns with the relationship between my performance and appearance and my value as a person.

My preoccupation with self-image dictated that I had a lot of face to lose. I had been in clinical management positions that imbued me with status, responsibility, and authority since 1989. Consistent with a lifetime's worth of messages and conditioning, my professional roles were fundamental to my sense of self.

Tucson is a beautiful Southwestern city situated in the high Sonoran Desert at an elevation of 2,000 feet, surrounded by four different mountain ranges with some peaks exceeding 9,000 feet. It is the second largest city in Arizona, and in spite of a population of approximately 500,000 (in the mid-2000s), the city retained the feel of a small town.

The local network of behavioral health and social services providers was a considerably smaller community. There were an impressive number of interagency collaborations. Our agencies were partners in some programs and contracts to provide services, and competitors for others. A multitude of meetings for planning, resource allocation/coordination, and service delivery were attended by many of the same professionals representing the same agencies—the usual suspects, as I referred to them. It was an incestuous fraternity where most everyone knew most everyone, particularly at the higher administrative levels.

Saving face in the context of addiction takes on outsized importance due to the stigma attached to it—both public (external) and self (internal). Public stigma—how addicts are viewed and treated socially—includes stereotypes based on negative beliefs, i.e., they're dangerous, weak of character, etc.; prejudiced attitudes that discredit and devalue addicts based on agreement with those negative beliefs; and discrimination in the form of behavioral responses to that prejudice, such as limiting funding for treatment and other supportive services, and so forth.

Self-stigma involves taking the same kinds of stereotyped negative beliefs that society has about addicts and applying them to oneself on a personal level. I believed that if I was an addict, then I must not only be weak, but fundamentally "bad." By internalizing those negative self-perceptions, I discredited and devalued myself, cratering my self-esteem and sense of personal self-efficacy. My self-stigma energized the shame that animated those long ago, yet not-so-far-away issues from childhood, and had me holding on to my face tenaciously—as if for survival—contributing directly to my failure to seek help.

To me, admitting my addiction and seeking treatment meant losing face, and losing face meant suffering public disgrace and the loss of an essential part of my identity. To avoid this fate, I *had* to save my face; I *had* to hold on to it! What did I have, if I didn't have my professional face? As I would learn from my first sponsor, Phil, this was a function of the self-centered, fear-based thinking intrinsic to my addiction. In my obsessive need to hold on to my face, I ended up losing my ass.

Active addiction is a relentless deviation-amplifying system—a system that over time throws itself further and further out of balance. Take the weathering of rock, for example. It begins with a tiny crack. A small amount of water collects in the crack. The water freezes and the force of the ice it forms enlarges the crack in the rock, however slightly. The larger crack collects more water, which makes the crack still larger when it freezes. The process continues—the growing crack collects greater amounts of water that freezes, increasing the size of the crack until it breaks the rock altogether, shattering it into pieces.

chapter eight

[CRISIS CREATES OPPORTUNITY]

"One of these days I'm gonna pull myself together
Soon as I finish tearing myself apart."
JOHN BARLOW, *GENTLEMEN, START YOUR ENGINES,* GRATEFUL DEAD

Neuroscience demonstrates that repetitive experiences involving substances (or activities, such as gambling, eating, sexual involvement, video gaming, spending, etc.) have profound effects on the brain's structure and functioning—effectively taking over its reward system and contorting priorities to enable their continuation. Over time, the capacity for conscious choice dissipates, and with enough repetitions effectively disappears. Addiction in all its forms includes the loss of voluntary control and a vicious cycle of repetitious and self-defeating behavior.

Each new strategy to self-manage my opioid pain meds crashed and burned on takeoff. All I wanted was to find a way—any way—to make them last long enough to get me to that magic thirty-day threshold when I could re-up my scripts. And I just couldn't do it. Even though *this* month, *this* time, *this* strategy was going to be different damn it; with the consistency of a high-end Swiss watch, every single attempt to control my using collapsed as soon as it was implemented.

As the cracks in my edifice of self-deception grew larger, I began to feel increasingly despondent, demoralized, and desperate. There are numerous theories on the etiology of depression, one of which is the psychoanalytic view that it represents anger turned inward against the self. I began to despise myself for having allowed my using to steal my emotional availability from my family and to commandeer my life as it had. I was helpless and hopeless in the face of its demands for care and feeding, as if it were a hijacker that assumed control of the airplane and I was the fucking flight attendant.

It wasn't supposed to happen this way. I was a professional—drug user, that is. I knew how to do this; I had done it for so long. Reality without some degree of mood- or mind-alteration was strictly for those rank amateurs who couldn't handle drugs. For someone who had always prided (and later deluded) myself on having my shit together while being able to continue using, this was an especially breathtaking failure. I had never failed so completely at anything. The ripple effects of this failure intensified as the consequences of my addiction-driven actions steadily piled up and my outward functionality continued to implode.

However strong a swimmer I thought myself to be, I was being pulled under and swept away by a riptide for which I was no match. I had always clung to the belief that if I just swam smarter and harder I could stay ahead of it. After so many years of swimming against this current, I came to the point where I was swimming as fast as I could and still getting dragged farther and farther out to sea, watching the shore and my connection to it grow fainter.

The inexorable truth the phenomenon of tolerance teaches all addicts is that the longer they use (regardless of the substance), the less of the desired effect they will experience from the same quantity. As human biochemistry adapts to the substance and becomes used to it, it takes more of that substance to produce the same mind- and mood-altering effects. One of active addiction's cruel realities is that gradually and progressively, the drugs work less and less well. The only options are to continually increase the amount used or to switch to a more efficient route of administration that delivers the payload more rapidly—such as smoking or shooting—to the brain's reward center; however, even these are but temporary fixes. If we use long enough, the dope basically stops working and only serves the purpose of keeping the agony of acute withdrawal at bay.

The drug-induced dynamics of diminishing returns have two levels: micro, which is declining effects with each successive dose over the course of a day, and macro, which includes decreasing desired effects that occur over the total length of time one has been using, whether weeks, months, or years. As the years progress, addicts in active addiction continue to chase the sublime intensity of the high, the buzz, the rush they experienced early in their using careers. Addicts retain vivid Technicolor memories of that revelation of chemically induced ecstasy, romanticizing the hell out of it. It is that perfect moment, resplendent as the recollections of one's first true love. It is the addict's solemn, dedicated mission to recapture that pure, unspoiled essence.

At a certain point in my evolution as an addict, I stopped getting high. Past that threshold, I used drugs just to feel what had become for me "normal," and to avoid getting sick. It had long since ceased being fun, and had become another form of work—a job unto itself. The toll of my increasing tolerance to opioids had turned my oh-so-familiar-blissful-pain-numbing-water-off-a-duck's-back-everything-is-okay-warm-fuzziness into a frustrating and futile quest for that Holy Grail. The relief from my pain and stress had become momentary at best. But did that dissuade me from chasing the next dose on the possibility that this one would be, could be, better?

I *knew* that delicious euphoria was still there—somewhere—it fucking had to be! The reality was that after more than eight years of daily use, the equivalent of overfishing those waters had rendered what I was searching for all but extinct.

To add insult to injury, the torment of my monthly self-detox was only getting worse, holding me hostage to my bed and bathroom, while I missed work that required the presence and attention I couldn't give. For the first few years, I was able to tough it out and drag my ass to work, but my withdrawal symptoms became progressively more severe in acuity and duration, and I began to miss one to two days each month. I had plenty of sick time available and played off my absences by claiming this or that illness, with acute back pain as an ever-available possibility.

My supervisors, supervisees, and other coworkers were generally aware that I had a chronic pain condition for which I took opioid medications. No one ever expressed suspicion or suggested that I might be an addict, at least not to me—with a single exception. After the incidents that would bring me before the AZBBHE came to light, my supervisor at JFCS, the CEO, asked me if I had a substance abuse problem. I deflected this inquiry with the explanation I would later use with the AZBBHE, that my chronic pain had lamentably led me to exercise poor judgment and decision-making.

Unlike going cold turkey from alcohol, benzodiazepines (such as Valium, Xanax, and Ativan), or barbiturates (like Seconal, Nembutal, and Tuinal), no one is at risk of dying from opioid withdrawal; it just feels like you are going to die, and the experience was so torturous that sometimes I wished I would.

Occurring every month as it did, it was like my very own menstrual cycle. And with it came my monthly attempts to convince my wife that this time I was legitimately sick.

"No really, this time I have some kind of flu bug."

She had gotten to the point where she would respond with a disgusted and matter-of-fact directness.

"Bullshit, you're out of meds and you're going through withdrawal again."

It was pathetic. I was pathetic. And I had a burgeoning sense of being irreparably broken.

Always a possibility lurking in the back of my head was that I could supplement my opioid pain meds with heroin bought on the street. Tucson is just sixty miles north of the international border with Mexico, and it was well known that heroin was easily available and inexpensive on the south side of the city. The behavioral health and addiction-related programs I administered served many addicts well-versed in the wares of the South Tucson marketplace.

With all the lines I had already crossed and all of the serious risks I had taken, I couldn't bring myself to seriously consider that option. There were excellent rational explanations, not the least of which was that if my random urinalysis came up positive for heroin, my social work license would be history—and I wasn't willing to give up on it at that point. However, the decision-making that occurs under the influence of active addiction has little connection to rationality. In hindsight, as lost and as ethically and spiritually bankrupt as I was, I believe that part of me knew if I crossed that threshold and returned to using heroin, I'd lose my soul in such a way that I might never find it again.

I couldn't continue using painkilling opioids the way I had been, but I couldn't stop. I was trapped in this double-bind and didn't see a way out. But something *had* to change. Active addiction is often thought of as a gradual and indirect form of suicide. For the first time since I was an adolescent (when it is not all that uncommon for teenagers to contemplate it to one degree or another), I began to consider the possibility of offing myself. As I wandered the fast track of definitive self-destruction, I couldn't fucking believe that I could ever get to *that* place, yet here I was.

The irony that I had performed suicide assessments on many clients and trained dozens of therapists in how to conduct such assessments was not lost on me. Once suicidal ideation (thoughts of committing suicide) is present, four basic areas must be explored in assessing suicidal potential:

1 Does the person have an actual plan to kill him- or herself? If the person has a plan, how specific is it?

2 How potentially lethal is the plan? In other words, if the person carries out his or her plan, how likely is it to be fatal?

3 Does the person have access to the means to carry out his or her plan? For instance, if the plan involves a gun, does the person have access to one? If the person doesn't have immediate access to the means to carry out the plan, how easily could he or she get it?

4 How committed is the person to acting on his or her plan? To what extent does he or she fully intend to follow through on it and attempt to take his or her own life?

These questions comprise a continuum of severity and risk—the more of them that are answered in the affirmative, the higher the degree of danger for the person in question. I observed myself with a perverse, morbid bemusement—in a depersonalized sort of way, as if watching myself from outside my body—making progress toward increased risk and potential lethality.

• My suicidal ideation became more coherent and serious. Check.

• My plan was that I would go to South Tucson and buy a big enough package of heroin to ensure a fatal overdose, stick a needle in my arm for the first time in over two decades, push the plunger in all the way, and fade into oblivion as my respiration slowed to the point that my breathing stopped altogether, and go to sleep permanently (unless of course, I ended up puking and aspirating the contents of my stomach into my lungs, thus suffocating on my own vomit; less peaceful but equally effective)—a clear and specific plan. Check.

- My plan possessed excellent potential for lethality (I was not going to attempt to OD on aspirin or Tylenol—although taking acetaminophen in extremely high doses is toxic and can lead to liver failure). Check.

- I had access to the means to carry out my plan. Check.

In counseling in general, and addiction treatment in particular, one of the most basic and important responsibilities is to help clients access a glimmer of hope where there is usually so little, and then help them build upon that hope. I've always believed that facilitating a client's ability to see even a little bit of light at the end of a pitch-black tunnel was among the most valuable and therapeutic things I could do.

There are so many similarities between providing psychotherapy to clients and providing clinical supervision to therapists that they are often described as parallel processes. For me, a common parallel involved instilling hope in therapists working under my supervision that they had the capacity to be helpful to clients who were so damaged that they sometimes seemed hopeless and beyond all help. Often, the difference between hopelessness and ever-so-slight hope lay in a change in perspective. Many of the clients we worked with had extensive, often multigenerational, histories of abuse, trauma, addiction, acute and chronic health challenges, poverty, and emotional abandonment.

Given their life experiences, it wasn't surprising that they had the serious problems that brought them to us. Sometimes it is remarkable that people survive the various kinds of hell they endure. Just to survive these experiences requires considerable strength and courage. Such strength and courage represent resources that can be tapped and brought to bear intentionally, in the service of coping with and overcoming all sorts of challenges. Helping therapists identify their clients' internal resources and utilize them therapeutically made important and positive differences in the outlook of both therapists and clients. And yet, here I was, alone in the darkness of my own internal emptiness, without any semblance of hope for myself—just another heaping helping of irony.

In active addiction, the obsessive thoughts and compulsive behaviors that focus like a laser beam on accessing and using drugs precipitate an all-encompassing self-centeredness. It is a relentless, single-minded, and self-absorbed pursuit of one's own desires and perceived needs— including the increasingly elusive "rush" reminiscent of those first using experiences. The self-centeredness is so fierce, it can preclude any meaningful consideration of the needs of others, or the potential consequences of one's actions. The self-centeredness of my active addiction cultivated an attitude that demanded immediate gratification— getting what I wanted when I wanted it, which usually translated to right now, if not sooner.

This self-centeredness separates the addict from others and from the world, isolating him or her in a cocoon of narcissistic preoccupation. It is characterized as the spiritual component of addiction since spirituality requires a sense of connection to that which is outside of oneself. It involves experiencing a positive connection to other people, to the world around, and to powers beyond oneself—the universe; a higher power; the god of one's own understanding (which may or may not have anything to do with an organized religion), a feeling of belonging to a larger, greater whole.

Spirituality involves practicing the principles of faith and trust. However, during my active addiction, the primary ways I applied these principles was in maintaining faith that using would continue to change my feelings to suit my preferences, and trusting that the drugs would keep working as they had promised early on.

Suicide is a consummate act of self-centeredness. It is unmitigated narcissism in action, regardless of the depth of the emotional pain that drives one to it and regardless of the rationalization that those left behind will somehow "be better off."

The only element missing from my suicide self-assessment profile was a commitment to carry out my plan. What shook me from the spell of my active addiction's ferocious self-centeredness enough to keep me from acting on my plan was my love for my daughters, in combination with my professional knowledge of the nightmarish legacy that parental suicide leaves to the children left behind. Parental suicide is one of two factors placing people at the highest risk for suicide themselves (the other being previous suicide attempts on their own part). It haunts children throughout their lives and often sets them on the path for other self-destructive behaviors, including addiction.

This didn't make me a better or nobler person than anyone else who struggles with addiction. My awareness was a facet of my behavioral health background. My academic studies and clinical experience had given me a multilayered understanding of the extraordinary responsibilities parents have to help their children feel safe in the world—emotionally, as well as physically.

Having that knowledge was a double-edged sword. Usually it was it was a blessing that gave me a wealth of information and greatly expanded my awareness of how I could be a better parent. But with that came the self-imposed burden of a higher level of parental responsibility and accountability—I felt an obligation to be a *better* parent; I knew too much not to. As my addiction metastasized, so did my guilt and shame vis-à-vis my shortcomings (both real and imagined) as a parent.

Because I understood that parent-child interactions are so complex and psychologically charged, part of me accepted that no matter what I did as a parent, it would provide potential fodder for my children's future therapy. But this was entirely different. No matter how much I was suffering—there was a limit as to how much suffering I was willing to inflict on them. Whacking myself might have ended my own suffering, but it would have perpetuated theirs.

At the time my daughters were fourteen and nineteen years old—in the throes of middle and later adolescence. At those stages of life, the developmental challenges are especially complex. It is a time of great uncertainty and confusion related to rapid changes and shifting expectations: expectations kids have of themselves, expectations others have of them, and expectations they have of others. It is a period of transition, of trying to figure out who you are and how you want to be in the world. How parents are viewed by their adolescent children shapes the children's ability to develop a coherent, healthy identity and has myriad implications for the kind of adults they will become. Of course, I didn't want to hurt my wife any further either, but she was an adult who had already demonstrated world-class resilience throughout her life.

The active addiction that I had kept in a state of seemingly stable equilibrium, so carefully for so long, had morphed into something new and different—a state of *dis*-ease that gripped me by the throat, threw me to the floor, and put me in a sleeper-hold, squeezing tighter and tighter. The harder I struggled, the deeper I sank. Devoured by pain, I continued to seek solace in the substances of my destruction. My misguided, ego-driven attempts at control only submerged me more completely into the quicksand. And the further from the truth I got, the more distant I became from those I adored, who needed and deserved so much more than I was able to give.

As human beings we have a remarkable capacity for dealing with serious shit when it hits the fan. It is when difficult, challenging circumstances are perceived as insurmountable—when we find ourselves without the physical, mental, emotional, or spiritual resources to deal effectively with stressful events—that we find ourselves in crisis. A crisis can be any event or series of events that create an unstable, potentially dangerous situation affecting an individual, family, group, community, or whole society. All crises share several defining characteristics that include being unexpected, producing high levels of uncertainty, anxiety, and stress, and representing a threat (real or imagined) to those affected.

A crisis situation can revolve around a specific incident such as an earthquake, tornado, tsunami, an industrial accident, or a terrorist attack. A crisis can also be related to any substantial change in the events that comprise the daily life of a person and his or her closest significant others. Such circumstances consist of situations that are life-altering and include everything from medical emergencies, serious injury, and long-term illness, to crime victimization, to the loss of a job/career and/or extreme financial hardship, to active addiction that can no longer go unaddressed.

Personal crisis is a state of psychological disequilibrium (imbalance) that occurs when extraordinary events trigger extreme stress within an individual. But it takes much more than just an extremely stressful event to create a crisis. Crisis results when the individual interprets the event as a grave threat—physically, mentally, emotionally—to self and/or significant others, *and* their usual methods of coping are either not available or ineffective.

One by one, each and every one of my conscious and unconscious coping mechanisms that had kept me safe and warm and dry—my rationalizations, my minimizations, my intellectualizations, my continuous machinations and manipulations to control people and situations to generate outcomes favorable to the maintenance of my active addiction, the totality of my denial—all collapsed like a saturated earthen dam no longer able to hold back rising flood waters.

Under the cloud of my social work license's probationary status, in July of 2005 I left JFCS after eight years to take a position as Regional Director at a well-known social and human services agency where my tenure was both mixed and brief. I had successes in writing grant proposals that were awarded funding and in composing the agency's first-ever behavioral health policies and procedures. But many staff (including those under my supervision) were in the throes of adjusting to multiple organizational changes, and I handled the resulting political and interpersonal challenges poorly enough that I was let go after ten months, albeit with a severance package of 25 percent of my annual salary.

The sudden uncertainty of our collective income led my wife and I to sell our beautiful home with a sixty foot lap pool and built-in hot tub with spectacular unobstructed views of the Santa Catalina mountains. I loved that house, and leaving it was a big loss. Although my wife was less enamored with it than I was, she was understandably angry and resentful that our move was coerced by my job loss. To make matters worse, we moved into a small, cramped apartment with obnoxious hard-partying neighbors.

Within six weeks I was hired as the Senior Director of Specialized Services for one of the three largest behavioral health service agencies in Tucson. I had worked on collaborative projects with the CEO previously, and he was delighted that I was available. The structure of my position made it difficult to manage under the best of circumstances, but in my increasingly impaired condition it was flat-out unmanageable. Nonetheless, with the addition of my salary, my wife and I were in contract to buy a house that we really wanted. When I was terminated after four months, the new house and our hopes for a better near future evaporated.

After nearly twenty years of professional success, I found myself unemployed and increasingly unemployable. Though no one at either of the two jobs I had lost in a fifteen month span ever expressed or even implied that substance abuse was the root cause of my problems at work, I knew better. As did my wife, who had had enough. My marriage of twenty-two years was hanging by a thin frayed thread.

Crises that challenge our perceptions of life-as-we-know-it and throw us into complete turmoil create substantial and meaningful opportunities for growth and change. Such opportunities may never have existed before, at least not in the conscious awareness of those caught in crisis.

As much as it didn't feel like it for me in those moments of flailing free-falling desperation, a process of transformation had already begun. The swamping of existing coping abilities makes clear that well-worn ways of thinking and acting are no longer sustainable.

This is especially true for problems like addiction, where intractable patterns of thinking, feeling, and behaving become deeply entrenched over time. Those caught up in crisis face an either/or dilemma: either adapt and develop expanded awareness and new coping skills or regress to lower levels of functioning. For addicts this translates to "either go on as best we can to the bitter ends—jails, institutions, or death—or find a new way to live."[9]*

Only a severe enough crisis could provide the motivation necessary for me to remove my head from the cramped but cozy confines of my ass after thirty years of using drugs in one form or another nearly every day. My options were unmistakable—there were only three, and I had ruled out two of them. I had to crawl through this shattered window of opportunity, dragging myself across shards of glass protruding from its frame and become open to new possibilities and willing to find a different way to live. It was the choice that felt like no choice at all, but it was the only viable option remaining for me—the one I had avoided for so many years: addiction treatment—fuck!

When I was a teenager, there was a TV commercial that ran in the metropolitan New York area for a particular brand of oil filter. This commercial featured a mechanic talking about people who bring their cars into his auto repair shop because they are not running quite right. Upon inspection, the mechanic informs them that their car needs an oil change and a new (insert brand here) oil filter. He continues, sometimes people just don't want to spend the money on a new oil filter. However, a year from now they might be bringing their car back to him—only this time, with major engine damage. By putting off paying the $20.00 for an oil change and new oil filter, they ended up with over $1,000.00 in engine

*(From *Narcotics Anonymous*, We Do Recover. Reprinted with permission from Narcotics Anonymous World Services, Inc.)

repairs. The mechanic looks directly into the camera and concludes, "The choice is yours: you can pay me now . . . or you can pay me later."

Avoiding facing certain problems gives the problems we wish to avoid time and opportunity to grow. Until I was ready and willing to address my active addiction, it was destined to fester like an untreated infection. Having been unwilling to pay earlier when the costs could have been considerably less, I was now confronted with having to pay a much higher price.

An easier, softer, and gentler path would have been nice, but that just wasn't going to work for me. I had to have my ass thoroughly kicked every which way before the pain of maintaining my active addiction exceeded my fear of doing anything significantly different. I had to receive the "gift of desperation" before I could become genuinely open to the possibility of meaningful change.

chapter nine

[VEGAS, BABY]

"Once in a while you can get shown the light
In the strangest of places if you look at it right."
ROBERT HUNTER, *SCARLET BEGONIAS*, GRATEFUL DEAD

I know that the god of my particular understanding has an excellent sense of humor because with all of the insane and crazy experiences I had had, the very first time I went to Las Vegas wasn't to celebrate or party my ass off or gamble . . . it was for addiction treatment.

Why Vegas, one of the world's epicenters of debauchery and Dionysian excess? When I was defeated enough to concede that I had to enter treatment for my addiction, the question remained, what about my chronic pain? What the fuck was I supposed to do about that? I had a legitimate diagnosed, long-standing chronic pain condition with the

MRIs to prove it. There were many things about going into treatment that scared the hell out of me, but what would become of my pain was high on the list.

Having spent half of my nineteen years of post-master's experience working in addiction treatment, I knew infinitely more about what was available and what to look for than the average consumer, but the addition of chronic pain to the equation complicated matters. It was late October of 2006. An Internet search yielded a grand total of three addiction treatment facilities in the entire US with dedicated chronic pain treatment programs. The only such facility west of the Mississippi was located in, of all places, Sin City.

The treatment center in Las Vegas was an abstinence-based twelve-step-oriented treatment program. At the time, I didn't necessarily want total abstinence or a twelve-step approach. There were programs out there that were not strictly abstinence-based and basically left the door open for using, especially when it was medically indicated. And there were plenty of programs that did not adhere to the twelve-step model. What was necessary was co-occurring treatment for my addiction and chronic pain, and with this priority ascendant, the choice of facilities made itself.

Once I begrudgingly accepted my need for treatment, by far the hardest thing I had to do was inform my daughters. I adore my kids. They touch places in my heart that no one else can reach. To paraphrase one of the Grateful Dead songs I used to sing to them as lullabies when they were very young, I love them "more than words can tell." I was soul sick at the prospect of how this might affect them—how they viewed and felt about me, and how they viewed and felt about themselves. Looking into their eyes and telling them that I was going to inpatient treatment for drug addiction was heartbreaking—for each one of us.

My older daughter was a sophomore at Arizona State University, living away from home. Her response evidenced the upset, pain, and confusion I so deeply dreaded. "What do you mean? You can't be a drug addict!

I've never seen you even close to drunk or messed up! You've always been there for us! We've always had nice houses and nice things. You've always had good jobs, and the bills always get paid!" Her words were testimony to my former facility in maintaining a double life, including the extent to which I had successfully kept distance between my children and the depth of my active addiction, and the resourcefulness of denial (in this case, hers).

The response of my younger daughter, who was just two months into her first year of high school, was much more muted, but no less pained. Wearing an expression of hurt and betrayal, she looked as though she wanted to cry but didn't. It was as if I could hear whatever remnants of parental idealization that had survived to that point in their adolescence breaking into tiny pieces.

I braced myself to enter treatment in the traditional way—I did everything I could to cram as much of what I loved into my body and brain as possible. Fortunately, I had recently re-upped my fentanyl script so I armored myself by ingesting two weeks worth of it in the three days leading up to my flight from Tucson to Vegas. When the staff from the Las Vegas Recovery Center picked me up at McCarran Airport, I was intently chewing one fentanyl patch and wearing three others. In addition to bracing for detox, I didn't want to leave any dope on the table—whatever I didn't use, my wife was going to dispose of, and that would just be wasteful.

Even at the very end, I never really wanted to stop using. Like the vast majority of people struggling with addiction, part of me held tight to the fantasy that somehow, it was still possible to find a way to control it and use "successfully." At the age of forty-seven, after using for well over three decades, the idea of giving up drugs altogether was like losing a limb to me.

As the combination of active addiction and chronic pain progressively took over my life and I saw the world as if through a tunnel, the losses I suffered grew in number and significance. Significant loss occurs whenever someone (family, loved ones, or friends) or something that has been meaningful in our lives is no longer available to us due to death, injury/illness, or the end of (or a substantial change in) a relationship. My ability to be physically active and participate in sports; my capacity to be fully emotionally available to my wife and children; my ability to maintain a "normal" mood and find pleasure; my health; my sense of self and self-esteem; my career and even my ability to work, as well as many of my hopes and dreams for the future—all deteriorated, morphing into losses of what once was.

Recovery creates the potential to regain many of the important things that are lost during active addiction. However, there is one loss that the recovery process requires without exception—the loss of the substances upon which addicts have depended so much for so long.

This particular loss tends to be under-recognized and grossly underappreciated—by those entering recovery in addition to those around them, and sometimes even by treatment professionals. Most people assume an attitude along the lines of "Good riddance! You're so much better off without that shit. Now you can get your life together." What is typically missed or minimized is the reality that this is a huge and painful loss, one that leaves a gaping hole in the lives of most addicts.

Even if one has reasonably healthy primary relationships, substances become a best friend, a lover, close confidante, and constant companion. For many people, active addiction was the most (in some cases, the only) intimate relationship they had. The impact of this loss is not to be underestimated. It smacked me upside the head mercilessly as I sleepwalked through the admission process that would formalize my transition from treatment program administrator to treatment program client.

Since I had shared my professional background with LVRC prior to my admission, the staff there was prepared for me to be a special challenge. Treatment professionals can be notoriously difficult clients in the same way that doctors can be among the most difficult patients. Up to this point, my professional knowledge and experience served to mobilize my denial, minimization, intellectualization, and rationalization—the defense mechanisms that had protected me from too much conscious contact with the depth of my addiction. Having once upon a time been in charge of the clinical operations of a hospital-based detox and rehab program, I was expected to be (as I would later learn from staff) a major pain in the ass.

After using powerful narcotics every day (except when I ran out) for eight long years, as well as having a truckload of fentanyl coursing through my system when I arrived, I needed to go through detox. Although I was hardly looking forward to this process—given that it culminates in being drug-free, an alien status I dreaded—at least it would be medically managed and include medications to keep me kind of, sort of, comfortable physically. I figured that had to beat the shit out of the agony I endured during my monthly adventures in self-detoxification.

I was quite familiar with medical detoxification protocols. Generally, the centerpiece of the medications used for opioid detox is a muscular opioid (most often methadone or buprenorphine) administered in dosages that successively get smaller—from some, to a little, to none. This was the lone aspect of the detox process I awaited eagerly; at least I'd get to use my dope of preference for a little bit longer en route to having to give it up. I could ease into its actual loss gradually, savoring those last few toned-down tastes of euphoria.

But it wasn't to be. The six days I spent in detox were a blur; not because the time went by fast, but because I couldn't see straight for most of it. And it wasn't because I was high . . . at all . . . damn it. Six different medications created a synergy that literally clouded my vision. And the only opioid among them was Darvocet, the weakest of all the opioids, and only a tiny amount at that—how fucking disappointing. And yet, to my absolute astonishment, I experienced none of the usual withdrawal symptoms and no acute discomfort!

The discomfort arrived with blunt force after I completed detox and relocated to the rehab side of the treatment center. During detox I actually slept well, but once off all medications, I didn't sleep for four entire days. It was brutal; I was an exhausted and empty shell, wondering when or if I would sleep again. Thank god for Dave, a twenty-one year-old recovery tech with eighteen months of recovery who worked the overnight shift. He was just a kid, but he hung out with me all night for four straight nights, displaying a wisdom and generosity of spirit far beyond his years.

When we are waist deep in the muck of a particularly intense thought pattern, emotional reaction, or physical sensation, that experience can feel as though it will last forever. I consulted with Dr. Mel Pohl, the medical director and detox magician. Dr. Pohl suggested that based on the frequency and duration of my using, it could be one to two months or longer before I returned to anything approximating a regular sleep cycle. My response: "You've got to be fucking kidding me." I later learned that Dr. Pohl is one of the foremost experts on chronic pain and addiction in the US.

I began to get a clearer sense of how dramatically my using had altered my biochemistry—up was now down. For the first week I cried openly, awash as I was in guilt, shame, and fear. Anxiety, regret, and sadness tossed me around like the imposing Atlantic Ocean waves I body surfed as a kid at Jones Beach on Long Island's south shore, flipping me ass over head and slamming me into the sand leaving me dazed, disoriented, and gasping for breath.

In individual sessions and groups I began to unmask myself, sharing my history of drug use, abuse, and addiction, in all its gory, twisted detail, with greater openness and honesty than I had ever been able to mobilize. With all the heartache and suffering I inflicted on myself and those closest to me on the road to getting my ass here, I figured I had damn well better make the most of it. To have any real chance of getting better, I knew I had to relinquish my natural inclination toward self-protection and control, and lay myself bare.

The chronic pain program was a revelation, providing state-of-the-art education on the science and dynamics of pain, including the phenomenon of opioid-induced hyperalgesia. Paradoxically, using increasing amounts of opioids over an extended period of time can actually cause more pain. The meds don't merely lose their effect—they trigger a syndrome of hypersensitivity to pain, even to stimuli that the body previously had not registered as painful. The only effective treatment for this condition is discontinuing opioid medications so the brain can "recalibrate" and eliminate the hyperalgesic effects.

I experienced a diverse array of holistic therapies, including assisted stretching, targeted chiropractic, acupuncture, massage, chi kung (sometimes spelled qi gong), yoga, Reiki, and physical therapy techniques I had never even heard of. Concentrated exposure to this comprehensive range of therapeutic modalities helped to accelerate my healing process, reducing my pain while increasing my functioning. It also gave me the opportunity to get a clear sense of which of these modalities best met my needs.

Chi kung proved to be an excellent fit for me; yoga and Reiki, not so much. A precursor to tai chi, chi kung is a moving meditation and gentle form of exercise that enhances the mind-body connection. It can lessen pain by releasing negative energy and restoring internal/external balance. In yoga practice, I strained my back, injuring it acutely, so that was a nonstarter. Reiki seeks to improve the flow and balance of energy by transmitting healing energy through the hands of the practitioner without actually touching the client. It was relaxing, but overall underwhelming to me.

There was one way in which Reiki was notable however. During one of my sessions, the practitioner was working with my energy when she described seeing the distinct image of a book. She was excited by this, saying that in her many years of Reiki practice she had picked up a wide variety of images from her clients' energy, but this was the first time she had ever seen a book. When I asked how she would interpret that, she asked if I had ever written a book. I told her I hadn't. She then said that the image could be about my education and its meaning for me, but she believed it meant that I would write a book (go figure).

In addition to physical interventions and techniques, treatment included changing the ways in which I think about my pain and react to it. I began to apply my preexisting awareness that chronic pain is a bio-psycho-social experience that has distinct biological/physical, psychological/mental, and social/cultural components. The biology of pain is a signal that "something is wrong" with my body; the psychology of pain is the interpretation or meaning I give to that pain signal—in other words, my beliefs about it; and the social aspect of pain is the way in which others, including family, friends, and medical providers react to me with regard to my pain condition—e.g., the degree of attention and sympathy I get. There is also a fourth dimension of impact: pain that is chronic also has spiritual manifestations. The spiritual aspect of chronic pain relates to my capacity to accept it as part of my total life experience rather than fighting against it.

Extending this bio-psycho-social-spiritual approach to pain, I was introduced to the beginning strains of a new concept: pain recovery. The basis of pain recovery is giving up the quest to be completely free of pain. The goal is to learn ways to accept the existence of pain, and how to coexist with it, rather than "kill" it. I began to develop the awareness to distinguish between my actual pain and the suffering created by it. Suffering results from mental and emotional reactions to pain. I started to practice and apply new skills to better accept my pain as well as find relief from that suffering. Adjusting the thoughts and beliefs I had about my pain effectively changes my emotional reactions to it, and that in turn, influences my actual experience of pain.

As arrogant as it might sound, even as an addict in inpatient treatment, I believed there wasn't much LVRC could teach me about drug addiction. Hell, I had been certified in Substance Abuse Counseling in both New York and Arizona, served as the clinical director of two inpatient addiction treatment facilities, and had taught courses on substance abuse as an adjunct professor at a small liberal arts college. I came to treatment steeped in knowledge about addiction—its dynamics, effects on the individual and family, treatment methods, relapse prevention, and current science/research. Plus, I had no small amount of personal experience to fit into my professional frame of reference. I had little need for in-depth education on addiction.

What I did not have was any understanding of recovery. Even though I had presented lectures on recovery to clients and had trained therapists on how to help facilitate their clients' recovery, whatever knowledge I may have had in this area was entirely intellectual. I had no clue as to how to stay clean myself. And as daunting as the task of not using seemed, I couldn't even imagine regaining a life of quality.

Prior to admitting my total defeat and seeking treatment, I dabbled briefly in SMART—Self-Management and Recovery Training, a self-help approach to addiction recovery. Based on the work of Albert Ellis, PhD, a psychologist who developed Rational Emotive Behavior Therapy (REBT), SMART uses the methods of REBT and Cognitive Behavioral Therapy (CBT) to focus specifically on the mental aspects of addiction. The emphasis is on identifying and trying to correct the faulty patterns of thinking and the distorted and irrational beliefs that contribute to the addictive process. According to the SMART program, rational thinking is the key to recovery.

My involvement in SMART was merely another strategy to avoid taking responsibility for my addiction and to forestall entering treatment. The handful of SMART meetings in Tucson were held at agencies that I had collaborated with professionally on several projects. My ongoing efforts to protect my "face" prohibited in-person attendance at those meetings— someone might recognize me and then I'd have to do some serious explaining. Determined to find the easiest option available, I attended a handful of online meetings SMART offered. I put little effort into this process and received little of value in return.

Nevertheless, I came to treatment armed with materials from the SMART program that I hoped to be able to pursue as an alternative to attending twelve-step meetings and doing "step work." Although most of the addiction treatment settings I had worked in had been twelve-step-oriented, and I knew that more people found and maintained recovery through twelve-step programs than any other method—by far—I came to my own treatment believing that it wasn't the right fit for me. (I was still operating under the illusion that my professional background somehow made me "different.") SMART was more consistent with my professional self-image, and my experience with CBT, as well as my need to keep the focus in my head where I was most comfortable. And for all my newfound openness and willingness, I was still trying to exert some control over my circumstances.

Prior to arriving at LVRC, I had attended a grand total of one twelve-step meeting, and that was an assignment for a class on substance abuse during my MSW program in 1986. Unlike most inpatient treatment centers that might take clients to one or at most two off-site twelve-step meetings weekly, once out of detox, clients at LVRC were taken to five outside meetings per week. In the face of my resistance to twelve-step programming, the staff could have easily said, "Tough shit, this is our approach. Take it or leave it."

Instead, my counselor referred me to Paul, the counseling supervisor who was initially taken aback by my request, but agreed that if I attended a full week's worth of twelve-step meetings and still had a problem with it, I could continue (start, really) with SMART. This was too reasonable to argue against; there was nothing for me to oppose. It was an aikido-like response that graciously presented me with structured options and allowed me space to find my own way without feeling coerced.

The extraordinary and genuine warmth of the welcome I received during my first twelve-step meetings was striking. It reflected a depth of unconditional acceptance that I had never experienced on a group level. At the second meeting I attended I heard a man with twenty-nine years of continuous recovery exclaim, "NA won't open the gates of heaven so you can get in, but it will unlock the gates of hell so you can get out." A switch was flipped, and for the first time I began to get the sense that maybe I wasn't as different as I thought I was. With an ease that took me by surprise, I traded the head-based method of SMART for the heart-felt and spiritually centered embrace of the twelve-step approach to recovery.

One of the unique aspects of LVRC is that the majority of staff are in recovery from addiction themselves—many of them for ten to thirty years. In the addiction treatment settings I had worked in professionally, 30 to 50 percent of the staff was in their own recovery. At LVRC this percentage was much higher, perhaps 70 to 80 percent. While the recovering staff I worked with previously would sometimes self-disclose and talk about their personal recovery, this technique was only used selectively, in specific situations. The staff at LVRC openly discussed their own recovery, routinely using it for purposes of example and role modeling in a much less clinically conventional way.

Moreover, almost all of the staff participated actively in a specific twelve-step program. They not only believed in this model of recovery, they lived it. I came to treatment needing more than anything else to learn how to live life without using drugs, and I was surrounded by living, breathing examples. If it worked for them, maybe, just maybe, it could work for me.

Inpatient treatment creates an incredibly intense environment. When it works well it provides a therapeutic milieu—a group setting that combines elements of support, structure, repetition, and consistent expectations to produce a physically and emotionally safe and trusting environment. Such an environment can expedite healing in several ways. It gives clients respite from the demands and stresses of their daily lives, providing a concentrated opportunity to focus on getting better. Clients feel comfortable enough to take the healthy risks of discussing deeply held secrets and experiment with healthy behavioral changes.

By exposing clients to each other's struggles, the milieu also facilitates mutual support and identification. This can help build connection, compassion, empathy, and understanding; reduce feelings of isolation; and generate new ideas and potential solutions regarding the challenges that brought them to treatment.

The other side of this coin is the increased levels of stress, anxiety, and upset that are commonplace when clients receive treatment in the same physical space where they reside twenty-four/seven, fenced in by an independence-inhibiting structure with foreign rules and expectations. The interpersonal dynamics and interactions between staff and clients, and among clients, are often highly emotionally charged. Factor in clients who are steeped in the drama and trauma of active addiction, all of whom are either going through detox or are just out of it, when they are at their most raw and vulnerable, in addition to some who are struggling with co-occurring physical and/or psychiatric challenges, and the environment can easily become superheated.

To say that addicts struggle with delaying gratification should be an obvious understatement. We generally don't respond well to not getting what we want when we want it. From a personality perspective, we are typically rebellious and oppositional; uninterested in adhering to rules and other social conventions, believing them to apply to other people rather than to ourselves. Disrespect for rules/laws ranges from the extremely serious to the minor who-really-gives-a-shit variety (as an example of my ongoing flouting of certain rules with which I disagree, I continue to enjoy jaywalking). Not surprisingly, many people have difficulty following the numerous rules inherent to inpatient treatment.

Some people end up leaving treatment prematurely "against medical advice." Others find themselves "administratively discharged" for violating red-line rules, such as bringing drugs on-site, physically fighting with other clients, becoming aggressive or threatening toward staff, or having sex with another client. Behavior that compromises the physical or emotional safety of the environment threatens the therapeutic value of treatment for everyone who shares that environment. As the clinical director of inpatient addiction treatment programs where I used to work, I was directly involved in the administration of limit-setting and discipline. When it came to problematic client behavior, my role was reminiscent of an assistant principal in high school.

At LVRC, I watched as some of my peers arm-wrestled with staff about this or that program rule or expectation. I was informed by another client that two of our peers had been placed on a behavioral contract due to concern that they had developed an "inappropriate" relationship. I heard about or observed various other forms of acting out, and it occurred to me that in my previous life I would have been responsible for addressing these kinds of situations—before I traded my private office with a large desk for a semi-private room with a bed and shower.

The process of preparing for discharge from most inpatient addiction treatment programs usually includes a group ritual during which all clients share their impressions of and experience with the person being discharged. Such groups are designed as a structured opportunity for formal good-byes, as well as to provide positive feedback and constructive criticism that the person being discharged can take with him or her as preparation for life outside treatment. In my professional addiction treatment experience, I sat in on dozens of these farewell-feedback groups and conducted quite a few of them myself. More often than not, they became a forum for emotional good-byes, superficial compliments, and clichés of encouragement. Among the most overused and least helpful remarks I heard with nauseating consistently were "You know what to do," and "I know you'll make it."

Really? I invariably reacted to the first statement by validating the importance of knowing what to do while emphasizing the Pacific Ocean-sized difference between that and actually doing it. As far as the second, it's natural for addiction treatment clients to want to believe that the peers whom they like and with whom they have bonded will be successful in continuing their recovery. This wishful thinking incorporates their hopes for themselves—if their friends "make it," so will they. But the reality is that most will not, at least not the first time around. This is not a reflection of the quality of treatment. The majority of people who receive treatment go through it without making a sustained post-treatment commitment to recovery.

When it was my turn to be the center of a discharge group at the conclusion of my stay at LVRC, the feedback I received was unanimously complimentary and well-intentioned. Many of my peers talked admiringly about my intelligence and how smart I was, as if this imbued me with some imagined immunity to relapse. When it was my turn to respond, I thanked them for their kind and generous words. However, I cautioned, my intelligence could be a curse as well as a blessing. It was an active ingredient in the processes of distorted thinking, self-deception, and manipulation of people and situations that buttressed my active addiction and enabled it to continue for so long. Intelligence in itself neither mitigates addiction nor facilitates recovery. It depends entirely on how that intelligence is used—it can be an asset or an enemy.

Treatment taught me far more than I ever knew about recovery as an ongoing journey of learning, growing, and healing. At the conclusion of inpatient treatment, many people believe they have completed this process. After what they've been through, and after all the effort they have expended, they want to think that they are finished and there is no more work to be done. This belief is natural and understandable, and although there are rare exceptions, it is usually mistaken. Fortunately, I knew enough to know better. My conscious awareness had transcended my intellect and begun to make its way from my head southward into my heart. My professional frame of reference had turned a corner and shifted from an obstacle to an asset on a level I could never have predicted. (Of course, I never would have predicted that I'd end up in addiction treatment "on the other side of the desk.") For me, the end of treatment was only the beginning.

The crucible of inpatient treatment is not necessary for everyone struggling with addiction. Plenty of people are able to get what they need, achieve abstinence, find recovery, and turn their lives around through outpatient treatment, other forms of counseling, and/or twelve-step program participation. My active addiction and its fusion with my chronic pain had reached the point where inpatient treatment was the only viable option for me. As much as I didn't want to be separated from my home and family for over a month, I was too far gone. I had lost too much of myself for a lesser level of intervention to have a realistic chance of being effective.

Whereas at earlier stages, treating an emerging addiction tends to be easier, less costly, and less disruptive, at later stages when severe adverse effects on major life areas are manifest, more intensive treatment is required. It's similar to taking care of a serious infection—painful, but necessary to facilitate healing and a return to health.

Suppose you get a small cut on your arm that for whatever reason was not disinfected with soap and treated with antibiotic ointment. The cut is no big deal and nothing to be concerned about in and of itself. However, because its proper care was neglected, it then becomes infected. The infection spreads so gradually that its existence and progression may not even be noticed. However, over time the cut becomes discolored, inflamed, and increasingly painful. You begin to feel weak and feverish as the effects start to impair other aspects of your health. At this point, the infection needs professional medical attention, probably treatment as an outpatient in a doctor's office.

If you continue to deny and minimize the infection's significance and avoid seeking treatment, it will continue to worsen, as the surrounding tissue becomes necrotic. Now, much more intensive medical intervention is required. Without it, gangrene may set in, necessitating amputation and potentially placing your life at risk. At that point, the infection must be effectively cut out through surgery, the entire area scraped clean and then treated with intravenous antibiotics. This process is costly, inconvenient, and painful. But without it, the infection will continue to progress, making recovery less possible, and premature death more likely.

Just prior to departing treatment, I met for a final time with Dr. Pohl to express my appreciation and discuss my aftercare plan, coordination of care issues for opioid-free pain management, and discharge summary (knowing that it would be required by the Arizona Board of Behavioral Health Examiners). He opened my medical record and showed me the picture that was taken upon my admission five short weeks earlier. I knew I felt absolutely horrible when I came in, but I had no idea that I looked even worse than I felt.

Dr. Pohl said, "Look at this guy. Look at how sad and depressed he is. And look at you now." I stared intently at the photo for a few long moments. My eyes were blank; my facial expression, zombie-like. I may have met the technical criteria for being alive, but inside I was lifeless. I couldn't help but smile at the contrast between how I looked then and the cautious optimism and reanimated hope I had begun to experience.

During my last four years on the opioid painkiller hamster wheel, every so often my prescribing doctor would ask me, "So, do you think you'll ever get off these opioids, or are you planning to stay on them for rest of your life?" I would always respond with a noncommittal answer along the lines of "I'll have to continue to see how my pain level is and what the options are," while inside my thoughts were *you bet your ass I'm staying on 'em; go ahead and sign me up for a lifetime contract.* I was playing for keeps.

Grief is a natural emotional state attached to loss. The conscious and unconscious suffering intrinsic to unresolved grief can contribute to both active addiction and chronic pain. Healing from grief involves mourning the loss to reach an acceptance of it. Mourning is a process of saying good-bye to, and letting go of, that which we have lost.

Achieving acceptance of a significant loss does not mean that there is no longer distress related to it. Losses that are fully accepted can still be painful, but they no longer create emotional imbalances that hinder health and healing. Much like a physical injury that has healed, there may always be a scar. Mourning and healing from grief is a process of regaining balance that takes time (months to years generally) and is different for each individual. This healing process requires that I allow myself to fully feel all the uncomfortable, painful emotions that are part and parcel of saying good-bye to and letting go of people and things that have been important in my life, but are no longer available to me. As the *Tao Te Ching* states in Verse 23:

> *"If you open yourself to loss,*
>
> *you are at one with loss*
>
> *and you can accept it completely."*

An important part of treatment for me was that it jump-started my process of mourning the loss of mind- and mood-altering substances. While I entered treatment resigned that I was probably going to "be forced" to stop using, I still had great trepidation and lots of ambivalence about giving up my primary coping mechanism. Almost no one comes to addiction treatment 100 percent voluntarily. Nearly everyone comes in with the aid of some form of coercion, be it external (legal, job-related, familial/marital/relationship) or internal (desperation, guilt, shame, or lack of other options). No one is happy about entering treatment, even if the person knows it's necessary and in his or her best interests. In this context, an abundance of ambivalence is natural and normal.

By the conclusion of treatment I had reached a place where I had fundamentally accepted letting go of my active addiction and came to terms with the need to mourn my loss of mind- and mood-altering substances. One of the very few positive effects of having used so much for so long and having used virtually everything every-which-way, was that I had left no stones unturned, no "research" remained to be done, and no questions left unanswered. I had demonstrated unequivocally to myself that I was constitutionally incapable of controlling my using. I had to accept the reality that I could no longer use, and begin to mourn that extremely significant loss.

The greatest emotional pain comes not from making meaningful life changes, but from mobilizing and maintaining resistance to such changes. After fighting against it for so long, in openly coming to terms with the reality that I was an addict, and had been since I was a teenager, I experienced a strange sense of liberation. I was so fucking tired of fighting. Eventually, attempting to control my addiction and its insatiable appetite for *more* became as absurd and as successful as trying to hold back the ocean tide. Consistent with the paradox woven into twelve-step recovery, ultimately I had to surrender to give myself any chance to win a war I had waged for three-quarters of my life—a war that was otherwise inherently unwinnable.

In order to begin the process of getting better and of healing, I had to admit complete defeat. In order to get my life together, I had to be done with tearing myself apart. This is the essence of Step One—to accept and admit my powerlessness over my addiction and the breadth and depth of the unmanageability it created in my life. In Buddhism, this dynamic is framed in terms of letting go of specific attachments—in this case, attachment to the need to deny that I was an addict and the belief that I could control my using and that I didn't need any help—as an essential ingredient in the lessening of suffering. Similarly, Taoism suggests that when two opposing forces meet in competition or battle, victory will go to the one that knows how to yield.

chapter ten

[ONE FOOT IN FRONT OF THE OTHER]

"The giant tree grows from a single seed.
A journey of a thousand miles starts
with the very first step."
TAO TE CHING, VERSE 64

Recovery consists of two basic parts: 1) getting "clean" (in the parlance of my twelve-step program)—discontinuing using, becoming abstinent, and halting the vicious obsessive-compulsive circle of active addiction; and 2) staying clean—remaining abstinent by learning how to live without using in an ongoing way. As hard as getting clean can be, this is actually the easy part in that it only has to happen once. Staying clean is much harder because it's a continuous, daily process. Mark Twain framed this distinction beautifully when he said, "Quitting smoking is easy, I've done it thousands of times."

As difficult as going through inpatient treatment can be, in some respects it's easy compared to the challenges of continuing the recovery process upon one's return to home and community. Quality treatment provides a sheltered, supportive, supervised, and safe (emotionally, as well as physically) milieu twenty-four/seven. The most arduous work in recovery commences upon one's re-entry into the "real world," outside of the protective cocoon of the treatment environment.

After completing treatment and coming home to Tucson, I struggled to adjust to life without using anything—no pain meds, no pot, no good red wine—absolutely fucking nothing. It was an alien planet and I didn't know how to be. I was in a constant state of withering physical and emotional *dis*-ease.

I felt so exposed, so raw. I flashed on long-submerged memories of an image from a March 21, 1969 *Life* magazine article that took my vision hostage in the waiting area prior to my then-weekly appointment with Dr. Gruber, the child psychiatrist I saw when I was in fourth grade. This image had been indelibly burned into my amygdala, the part of the limbic system in the recesses of the midbrain predominant in the formation and storage of memories associated with emotional and traumatic events. It was a picture of a baby seal that had just been skinned, during what was at that time an abhorrent annual ritual in a specific part of Canada by hunters who prized the coats of these very young seals. This baby seal was staring directly at me, still standing upright, covered in blood and completely stripped of its skin. Its coal-black eyes looked right through me. I wanted desperately to look away, and I couldn't.

A common misconception shared by many people, including those with addiction, their loved ones and friends, and even some less savvy medical and behavioral health professionals, is that very soon after the offending substances are out of the body (upon completion of detoxification or acute withdrawal), life will get noticeably better and "normal" functioning will return. If only that were true.

There are actually two distinct phases of the withdrawal process. Depending on the length and intensity of active addiction—that is, how frequently, how much, and for how long an individual has used substances, the second phase of the withdrawal process can last for weeks or even months *after* someone has stopped using. This exquisite phenomenon is known as post-acute withdrawal (sometimes referred to as protracted withdrawal), and I was savaged by a virulent strain of it. Post-acute withdrawal is a constellation of often brutally uncomfortable symptoms that persist after detoxification, after all physical traces of mind- and mood-altering substances have left the body and brain.

These symptoms affect many people in the early phases of abstinence from numerous substances, but occur in an extremely high percentage of those with histories of long-term opioid abuse. Post-acute withdrawal varies in intensity and duration from one person to another, again, usually in correlation with the intensity and duration of one's active addiction. Its manifestations can fluctuate in severity, coming and going in wave-like recurrences, and include impairments in energy, concentration, attention span, memory, sleep, appetite, and mood, such as irritability, anxiety, and depression.

Post-acute withdrawal is another consequence of the significant changes to brain anatomy and chemistry created by active addiction over the course of—in my case—three decades of using daily. The brain's reward system is turned on its head, and its natural ability to cope with stress is undermined. As long as I used opioids, my brain adjusted by decreasing its natural production of endorphins while increasing the number of opioid receptors, making it much harder for me to experience pleasure in the absence of using.

In early abstinence, the brain's stores of both endorphins and dopamine are severely depleted. Dopamine, the neurotransmitter that floods the brain during drug use to produce titanic highs, is also involved in the regulation of mood, and a certain amount of it is necessary in order to maintain a "normal" mood. The absence of this necessary threshold of dopamine creates a biochemically based depression. It can take weeks to months for the brain to naturally manufacture enough endorphins and dopamine to replenish its inventory of these vital brain chemicals.

The human nervous system consists of two main parts, the central nervous system (CNS) and the peripheral nervous system (PNS). The CNS contains the brain and spinal cord. The PNS consists mainly of nerves, long fibers that connect the CNS to every other part of the body so that information can be sent back and forth between the brain and the entire body. The autonomic nervous system (ANS) is part of the peripheral nervous system and acts as a control mechanism for most internal organs and ordinarily functions below the level of conscious awareness.

Active addiction precipitates a massive increase in the activity of the sympathetic division of the autonomic nervous system. The sympathetic division of the ANS is activated under circumstances of perceived threat and sets in motion the chain of physiological responses that prepare the body for "fight or flight." These unconscious responses automatically put mind and body on high alert, priming for action by initiating hypervigilance, increasing heart rate, constricting blood vessels, increasing blood pressure, dilating pupils, and inhibiting digestion.

Fight or flight mode kicks into gear in response to the stress of potential threats, but the nature of these physiological reactions themselves creates additional stress that becomes chronic in active addiction as the stress switch is stuck in the "on" position. This taxes the hell out of many of the body's systems, leading to a wired form of exhaustion, a run-down immune system, and greater vulnerability to illness, and yes, stress.

This chronic stress response continues during post-acute withdrawal, receding and effectively resetting only gradually over time. As a result, people come into recovery under the influence of biologically birthed higher levels of stress in combination with an enhanced susceptibility to stress. Meanwhile, early recovery can be incredibly stressful in and of itself. All sorts of stressful situations inevitably arise, and the frustration, confusion, and blistering discomfort of post-acute withdrawal symptoms (stress-inducing themselves) piggybacks onto them to produce even more distress.

Even though it's a driving factor in many relapses, post-acute withdrawal is often under-recognized and its impacts under-appreciated. Both addicts and their significant others are commonly encouraged to believe that as soon as the high cost of low living is relinquished, life will begin to improve rapidly. When reality fails to fulfill this unrealistic expectation, the disappointment is a bitch. It is not unusual for addicts in very early recovery to return to using, believing that "if this is what being in recovery feels like, screw it; I might as well use!"

In my early recovery I was buffeted by fatigue, restlessness, anxiety, irritability, depression, and sleep disturbances. I attended my first twelve-step meeting in Tucson on December 8, 2006, two days after returning from treatment in Las Vegas. I was thirty-four days removed from my last use of opioids, and I was an absolute fucking mess, still sleeping very little and irregularly.

I attended meetings every day for nearly six months. When I celebrated sixty days in recovery, I was still a mess—restless, irritable, and profoundly uncomfortable in my own skin. It was all I could do to put one foot in front of the other, get to a meeting every day, and since I was unemployed, mobilize the energy to put dinner together for my family. When I celebrated ninety days, I was still a mess—wracked with fatigue, anxiety, and depression. It wasn't until I had about 120 days in recovery—four full months since I had last used drugs—that I began to see some light at the end of the tunnel and feel a little more comfortable, physically, mentally, and emotionally.

This was another area where my professional background would prove to be an invaluable resource. Even though it felt as though it would last forever, I was aware that post-acute withdrawal is temporary. As nasty as its symptoms were for me, I knew eventually they would subside. Besides, I was also aware that if I returned to using, the blowback would include eventually having to go through acute and post-acute withdrawal all over again, as my brain and body went through the necessary process of rewiring themselves to adjust to living without drugs.

Abstinence is instrumental to healing the neurological impacts of addiction. It took around seven to eight months after my last use of drugs for the worst parts of my post-acute withdrawal to run their course. With the aid of neuroplasticity, the human brain has remarkable abilities to heal. Research using brain scans indicates that with about one year of abstinence, noticeable healing of the adverse changes caused by active addiction has taken place,[10] and with five years of abstinence, the brain often begins to resemble that of a person who has never used alcohol or other drugs. This notwithstanding, some addiction-caused changes will remain. The brain's reward center and the mesolimbic dopamine system that feeds it are forever altered.

Early recovery is full of serious challenges. Just in case the obstacle course of post-acute withdrawal isn't enough, let's add in the loss of one's primary method of coping with the world, along with the gift of experiencing—in all their glorious undiluted intensity—the uncomfortable feeling states that were previously blocked out, numbed, sanded down, and otherwise kept at a distance by using. Fortunately, feeling good is not a prerequisite for recovery.

While I stayed clean, I did a lousy job of balancing working on my recovery with being emotionally and physically available to my family. I had so little knowledge or experience of how to live without using mood-altering substances. A part of me knew that the only way I would have a chance was to dive headfirst into my twelve-step program. One of the great ironies of this time period was that because of the way I used, during my last eight years of active addiction, I was always home, even as my use of narcotic pain meds became increasingly beyond my control. I used at home, "jonesed" at home; I was around my family whenever I wasn't at work. I generally didn't want to go out or be with other people.

In contrast, after I got into recovery, I was away from home and my family much more than I had ever been—attending meetings and fellowshipping, getting to meetings early and staying afterwards to connect and spend time with like-minded folks to absorb as much of whatever I could learn from them as possible. A part of me knew that my best (perhaps only) chance to sustain recovery successfully was to stay in close contact with recovering people and resources, yet this created that much more conflict and stress at home.

My active addiction had perpetrated so much harm to my marriage, and there was an expectation between my wife and me that in recovery all would be well, and that I would repair the damage and be physically, as well as emotionally, available. It didn't work out that way, and in retrospect, as reasonable and understandable as that expectation seemed when it was established during family counseling sessions when I was in treatment, it may never have been realistic for me, at least during my first year in recovery. There was also an expectation that once in recovery, I would be a different person. I was—just not the person either of us anticipated.

I was unemployed for six months after treatment. The professional success I had enjoyed for so many years seemed irrelevant. I was seriously damaged goods. No one was going to hire me for the kind of clinical management positions I had held for over fifteen years, and I was thoroughly overqualified for the majority of job listings I replied to. I had been long accustomed to being invited to interview for a high percentage of the jobs I applied for, but I wasn't getting a sniff.

My struggle to find work in my field was complicated further by decisions I made pertaining to my professional credentials. I allowed my state substance abuse counseling certification to expire, believing that I had sufficiently demonstrated my lack of fitness to provide or oversee services specific to that arena (at least for the time being). After an agonizing process that encompassed consultation with several attorneys as well as other experts, and multiple unsuccessful attempts to arrive at a mutually acceptable alternative with the State Board of Behavioral Health Examiners, I also decided to surrender my state social work license.

These were crushing losses—I had had these credentials for many years—first in New York, and then in Arizona. They were required by state statute in order to provide psychotherapy, supervise therapists, and manage counseling programs. Earning and maintaining them in good standing had been among my highest professional priorities. And now they were history, added to my ash heap of wreckage, along with my ability to practice my chosen profession, and my carefully cultivated professional identity. Even in recovery, the casualties of my active addiction continued to mount.

After an extensive job search, I received two offers, one of which paid 25 percent more than the other. After considering the trade-offs, I accepted the lower paying position because it was much more supportive of the needs of my recovery, giving me greater opportunities to attend meetings, including my home group, which met every day (except Sunday) at noon. Having to choose between taking better care of my recovery and taking better financial care of my family, especially after my wife had been the sole income earner for half a year, presented a double-bind that I knew would cover me in crap one way or the other. Understandably, the choice I made only exacerbated the negativity and conflict between my wife and me.

The unfortunate statistical reality is that many long-standing marriages and other primary relationships don't survive the first year after one partner enters recovery subsequent to years of active addiction. Over time these relationships progressively adjust to the presence of active addiction, establishing a certain equilibrium. However inherently healthy recovery may be, it represents a dramatic change that throws this equilibrium completely out of balance. The required adjustments in relationship dynamics are severe, often exceeding the capacity and/or willingness of one if not both partners, regardless of how well-intentioned they may be.

I was barely treading water while trying to learn how to live without using, and after more than twenty-six years together and twenty-three years of marriage, my wife had had enough. Even though we had many more good years together than not, and had previously survived some serious challenges, the accumulation of everything we had been through, everything that I had put her through, proved to be too much. I couldn't help but agree with her that too much damage had been done, and our needs were moving in divergent directions.

Nine months after I returned home from treatment we decided to divorce. We had been together for more than half of my life, had raised two amazing children, and took real pride in being an intact biological family. It was a loss the scope of which is beyond words, replete with breathtaking sadness. I was unable to be what the competing, often seemingly conflicting needs of my circumstances demanded, and my marriage lost.

chapter eleven

[AN IMPERFECTLY PERFECT]
SUPPORT SYSTEM

"Maybe you'll find direction
Around some corner
Where it's been waiting to meet you."
ROBERT HUNTER, *BOX OF RAIN*, GRATEFUL DEAD

Just shy of celebrating my first full year in recovery, our divorce became final. It was as amicable as such a thing can be—we used one attorney and went through mediation, making a conscious and concerted effort to minimize animosity and be as cooperative as we were capable of being. In spite of our conflicts, we agreed that it was a fitting way to honor our relationship and what we had built together. Still, the process was far from easy and steeped in pain.

As we unwove the tapestry of our partnership, every thread we pulled, from the symbolic to the concrete, was another chunk of loss and one more opportunity to grieve. Strangely, it hit me hardest when we went to our long-time bank together to dissolve our joint accounts. We had always maintained joint accounts. Many married couples prefer to maintain separate bank accounts, but that idea had always seemed foreign to us. Since before we were married, our financial resources were continuously co-mingled. Sitting at the bank officer's desk, going through the process of closing our joint accounts and opening individual accounts evoked a sense of finality and opened up a new well of overwhelming sadness I didn't realize existed until that moment.

In spite of a fundamental acceptance about the divorce, I felt like I had failed, especially as it related to my daughters. During the last couple of years leading up to it, they had been through too much, and the past twelve months had been catastrophic in the life of our family. Knowing how divorce can affect kids, even adult children, only magnified my sense of guilt. And although they suffered as the arguments between my wife and I grew in frequency and fervor and the negativity became thick enough to spread on toast, the divorce irreparably altered the world as they had always known it, forever downsizing whatever sense of certainty and emotional safety they had.

In addition to all of the weight and complexity connected to the divorce, the residue of my post-acute withdrawal was still resolving, and my chronic pain (though improved even in the absence of opioid painkillers) sure as shit hadn't disappeared in the wake of my getting clean. A hurricane of mixed emotions swirled around me at what felt like ninety miles an hour. It would have been easy; in fact, it would have been natural and normal to get swept away in the stress of those gale force winds of change. And yet, that didn't happen. To my amazement, I was able to remain fairly centered and observe my sadness, anxiety, fear, and guilt in all their intensity, allowing myself to feel them without being consumed by them.

Given how much of my life as I had known it was in flux, the friends I had developed in my twelve-step fellowship expressed surprise that I didn't seem to be more crazed or freaked out. And somehow, how I felt inside was basically consistent with how I appeared on the outside. In asking myself, "How the fuck is it possible for me to be as okay as I seem to be?" the answer that emerged was surprisingly simple: I now had a program of recovery—a defined pathway toward health and healing—and I was making a concerted effort to utilize it as a resource and work it to the best of my ability.

I continued to find ways to integrate my twelve-step recovery with whatever understandings and skills I could mobilize from my professional life. The synergy that emerged allowed me to spend more time than not in the eye of the emotional hurricane—where stress-amplifying adversity and intensity spun at dizzying speed all around me, but I didn't have to spin with it.

As a psychotherapist and clinical administrator, along with many of my colleagues, I had long lamented that professionally provided treatment was often too limited in scope and duration, and as a result lacking in enduring efficacy. Inpatient and residential treatment, while providing care twenty-four/seven, lasts from mere weeks to a few months at most, and access to it depends explicitly on well-heeled individual financial resources, adequate health insurance coverage, or modest publicly funded services. Intensive outpatient treatment consists of combinations of individual, group, and family counseling for ten to twenty hours per week, usually for up to six months. Nonintensive outpatient treatment has the longest duration (up to a year or sometimes more), but the most circumscribed scope, between one and three hours per week of individual and perhaps group counseling.

Of course, professionally provided treatment is supposed to have an endpoint. The primary goal of any level of treatment should be to help clients progress to the point where treatment becomes unnecessary.

One of the criteria that defines success for treatment programs and providers is for clients to improve—in whatever area(s) of their lives brought them to treatment in the first place—enough so that they no longer need professional treatment, to effectively "graduate" from it.

But no matter how high quality the treatment services provided to clients might be; no matter how impressive the improvements they present in session are, it can be difficult at best to maintain those gains in the face of the stresses, strains, and dysfunctions embedded in many family, social, neighborhood, and work environments. The reality is that people naturally and appropriately spend much more of their daily lives in these environments than they ever will in treatment. The functional improvements clients make during treatment are mitigated if not undone through contact with these frequently countertherapeutic influences. This gooses the potential risk for a relapse of symptoms, or unhealthy behaviors—which, for anyone struggling to recover from active addiction, includes drug use.

Treatment providers regularly express the wish for an easily accessible and affordable community-based resource that can supplement professional treatment by providing social and emotional support, as well as a good enough "holding environment." Such a resource could provide clients with opportunities to consolidate and sustain the gains they've made, both between counseling sessions and after the conclusion of treatment.

The concept of the "holding environment" comes from D. W. Winnicott, the British pediatrician turned psychoanalyst. Winnicott viewed relationships and interactions with other people, along with how individuals saw themselves vis-à-vis their most important relationships, as the key factor in healthy development. He extrapolated his original holding environment—the physical and psychological relationship and interactions between primary caregiver (usually the mother) and infant child—to the relationship and interactions between therapist and client. Part of the therapist's task is to create a quality holding environment to assist the client's growth and development. The holding environment paradigm has since been applied to the family as a whole, in addition to other settings—such as school, recreational programs, church, synagogue, mosque, etc., and various social support systems—that surround us at any given point in our lives.

It didn't occur to me until I began my own recovery that twelve-step programs can provide that very resource. The holding environment of my twelve-step program gave me shelter from the heavy weather of my early recovery and supplied the support I needed to withstand its most extreme storms. A quality holding environment promotes feelings of physical safety and emotional security, of being understood and unconditionally accepted. It brings about such supremely humane and salubrious effects through consistency, reliability, attunement to one's needs, and by responding to those needs compassionately and empathically. By generating the experience of being emotionally "held" in these ways, this type of environment facilitates healthy physical, mental, emotional, and spiritual development.

A healthy holding environment gives to its occupants what Carl Rogers, the founder of Client-Centered Therapy, referred to as "unconditional positive regard"—the absolute, unequivocal respect for and appreciation of others encompassing such qualities as acceptance, nurturance, compassion, equanimity, empathy, and love. Being on the receiving end of unconditional positive regard, of feeling accepted for who one truly is, is a powerful cathartic. For those of us afflicted with addiction, it is an especially therapeutic experience.

Active addiction is one of the world's most effective ways of hiding who we really are. The stigma associated with it taints us and after a while we buy into it ourselves, magnifying our lack of self-worth. The longer and harder we use drugs, the more of our true self goes into hiding and remains hidden. We get further and further away from who we really are. The injuries we inflict upon ourselves and others multiply, and deep down we fear that we are inherently undeserving of the acceptance of others.

Consequently, for most of us the genuinely warm welcome, empathic understanding, and unconditional positive regard we receive in twelve-step programs of recovery is emotionally corrective. It offers a sanctuary that encourages us to take the healthy risks intrinsic to learning new and different ways of relating to ourselves and others, and grow beyond the boundaries of that which is familiar to us. It changes how we see ourselves, opening the door to self-acceptance. If others can accept me for who I am, even after I've bared the most carefully concealed parts of my persona and the worst things I've ever done, then maybe, just maybe, I'm worthy of acceptance and I can begin to learn to accept myself. Self-acceptance is essential in order to heal from the ravages of addiction.

The extraordinary acceptance I experienced in my twelve-step program was immediate and reflected a degree of unconditional positive regard that blew me away. That experience of acceptance without qualification continued as I transitioned to twelve-step meetings back in Tucson. Although there were some differences between the meetings in Las Vegas and those in Tucson, they were much more the same than they were different.

There are many individual differences among the people at any given twelve-step meeting: all the colors of the racial and ethnic rainbow; the entire socioeconomic ladder—from the homeless and desperately indigent to service workers and blue collar tradespeople to physicians, attorneys, and other affluent white collar folks; and the full educational spectrum, from high school drop-outs to PhDs and everything in between. In the case of my particular twelve-step program, the individual differences also include the complete gamut of so-called "drugs of choice," from street drugs (cocaine/crack, heroin/opiates, meth/speed, marijuana, hallucinogens), to those prescribed by a doctor (painkillers, tranquilizers, sedatives), or bought at a store like alcohol.

Addiction is a great equalizer, and a shared interest in recovery brings together this unusual assortment of people who would otherwise come in contact with one another only in passing. Somehow, the similarities that connect this diverse group of individuals overwhelm the vast differences between them. The commonalities we share: what we did in our active addiction—to ourselves, to our loved ones, and to others; the depths to which we sank en route to that place where we became sufficiently motivated to try to find a new way to live; our desire to remain free from active addiction; our challenges and struggles toward that goal, and faith in our twelve-step program as a pathway, to not only to achieve that goal one day at a time, but to learn how to live a meaningful and value-directed life—generate a deep connection that translates to empathic understanding and mutual support.

From the time I first started attending meetings in my twelve-step program, I felt at home. It is a simple program for people who tend to be complicated. Active addiction has a way of injecting extraordinary complexity into the ordinary events of everyday life. I may be complicated to begin with, but I also have the capacity to complicate the shit out of most anything. My usual way of complicating matters is by getting "stuck" in my head, falling into a sinkhole of rumination—obsessing, analyzing, and intellectualizing the hell out of whatever the issue might be. Step One of my twelve-step program makes no mention of substances or behaviors. Rather, it refers specifically to *addiction,* a disorder that manifests in obsessive thoughts, compulsive actions, and self-centered attitudes. Just because I became abstinent and entered recovery does not mean I became immune to these unhealthy ways of responding to the stresses and strains of life.

When I first started on the twelve-step path, all I was hoping for was to find a way to live free of the enslavement of the need to use drugs to control and change my feelings. What I found was that the Twelve Steps provide a structure with principles and tools to learn and practice how to live a whole, healthy, and healed life. To my further amazement, I discovered that the overall approach and cognitive-behavioral-spiritual principles of the Twelve Steps could be applied to my chronic pain with therapeutic effect.

At a meeting during my first few weeks back in Tucson, Anne, who had recently relocated from rural Virginia, shared in her lilting southern drawl, "If I don't pick up, I never have to 'jones' again." Her words smacked me upside the head. Holy shit, I never have to jones (go through withdrawals) again! On its face, this is self-evident, and intellectually I had always known it, but suddenly I truly understood it at depth, with all its implications. The realization that if I stay in recovery I'd never have to go through the torment of withdrawal again was a revelation. I have heard so many similarly simple sentiments in meetings that, along with the straightforward yet elegant wisdom of the sayings and much of the literature in my twelve-step program, bypass the analytical filter in my head and speak directly to my heart and spirit.

About a week prior to my discharge from the Las Vegas Recovery Center, my counselor and the client services manager (who at that time had eleven and twenty years in recovery, respectively) came to me saying, "We want to help connect you with a sponsor before you finish treatment." "How is that possible given that I live in Tucson?" I asked. They said that there was someone they knew well and had great respect for, who had been in recovery for nearly thirty years through the twelve-step program of which I was a newly minted member. They continued that this gentleman lived in the Phoenix area, and likely had experience with people in the program from Tucson and could potentially recommend someone as a sponsor.

A sponsor functions as a mentor or coach who helps guide people through the Twelve Steps and negotiate other aspects of recovery. In order to fulfill this role competently, he or she needs to have adequate experience in recovery and knowledge of working the Twelve Steps. Early on I learned that having a sponsor who is reliable, knowledgeable, and trustworthy is fundamental to the twelve-step recovery process, and an important part of one's support network.

I left Vegas with contact information for Phil, a fellow Tucsonan, who at that time had been in recovery for over twenty-three years. Although I started to attend meetings as of my second day back in Tucson, it took me a week to call Phil. It's freaky how heavy the phone can be at times. Phil's first words to me were, "I've been waiting for your call." Absent from his tone of voice was any hint of judgment or impatience; he was simply expecting to hear from me, and glad that we were now connecting.

He agreed to meet me later that day, at the meeting I had made my home group, the Midtown Nooners—we met at noon six days a week at the Quaker House, an old Victorian with magnificent natural interior light and an ample courtyard just west of the University of Arizona. Phil had grown up on the eastern shore of Connecticut, moved to Tucson in the early 1970s for college and stayed. We hit it off quickly, easily establishing positive rapport.

Among the ties that connected us—besides as he would say, addiction and recovery—were our Northeast coast origins, a love of sports, a passion for the Grateful Dead, and an appreciation of higher education. Many sponsors might have dismissed my professional background as either irrelevant or as an obstacle to my recovery. Phil made it clear from the beginning of our relationship that he viewed it as a strength that could complement our twelve-step work and enhance my recovery process. In fact, during one of our relatively early conversations, he told me that I would write a book that would encompass both my professional behavioral health knowledge and experience and my personal recovery.

Phil spoke in a gravelly yet soothing voice, and his face was accented most of the time by a beatific smile. He was unflinchingly gracious, kind, accepting, and generous of spirit. When I celebrated ninety days in recovery, Phil smiled broadly and said, "You know, the two hardest parts of recovery are the first ninety days . . . and the rest of it." When I celebrated six months he said, "You know, the two hardest parts of recovery are the first six months . . . and the rest of it." And when I celebrated one year, he looked at me knowingly and said, "You know, the two hardest parts of recovery are the first year . . . and the rest of it." His point was unmistakable: recovery is a never-ending journey, and life can throw difficult-to-hit pitches at us no matter how long we've been at it.

As I walked through the emotions of that fateful first year in recovery, Phil and I spoke at great length and in extensive detail about the wicked curveballs I faced. Sharing the unvarnished realities of your life with another person creates intimacy—a special, direct, and rich personal bond. Many people think of intimacy only in the physical sense; however, it extends far beyond that realm. Intimacy is about allowing someone else to see and get to know the true me. This can be a frightening proposition, especially for anyone who fears rejection or whose trust has been violated by people close to him or her—experiences in which most addicts are well-versed.

As humans we are social animals, hardwired for connection with others. Intimacy is an essential emotional need, and a cornerstone for building the capacity to have healthy relationships based on sharing and reciprocity. Intimacy with others is as important to emotional and spiritual well-being as food and exercise are to physical well-being. It is through the experience of speaking, being heard, and being understood with empathy and compassion, as well as being accepted exactly as one is, that we find self-acceptance. As Phil shared with me more than once, "The only thing any of us are perfect at is being imperfect."

I had been in recovery for a little over ten months when I had the privilege of tagging along with Phil to attend the celebration of the thirtieth anniversary in recovery for his sponsor, Billy. It was Billy who had recommended Phil as a sponsor for me when I was still in treatment in Las Vegas. I drove from Tucson to the festivities in Scottsdale with Phil and two other friends in recovery. Including my time in the program, there was nearly sixty years of accumulated time in recovery in our car.

Approximately 140 recovering addicts came from all over the Southwestern US and parts beyond to celebrate Billy's milestone of three decades in recovery through the twelve-step program we all shared. Most of those in attendance had at least fifteen to twenty years in recovery, many had twenty to thirty years, and some had even more. I felt like a minor leaguer who had been gifted with a pass to the New York Yankees clubhouse to witness a World Series championship celebration (minus the indiscriminate spraying of champagne). When I told that to Phil, he replied in his loving and relentlessly supportive way that, in his view, I was a major leaguer playing in my first World Series.

As speaker after speaker spoke about Billy's generosity of time, energy, and spirit, I got a compelling sense of some of the genealogy of our twelve-step program that was established as its own fellowship distinct from the parent of all twelve-step programs, Alcoholics Anonymous (AA) in 1953. Everyone in attendance had been affected by Billy in some extraordinary way. The sharing was in turns, poignant, laugh-out-loud funny, deeply spiritual, bittersweet, and awe-inspiring. One of his sponsees described those in attendance—as many as there were—as being only "the tip of the iceberg" of those whose lives had been touched by Billy. As many addicts whose lives he had touched directly and helped to change, each and every one of them had in turn touched the lives of many dozens of others, and so on.

And that is the way it is with this thing of ours. I feel as though I belong to a select and special club, and yet "the only requirement for membership is the desire to stop using." When it was the guest of honor's turn to speak, 140 people rose as one for a long standing ovation. His message was crystal clear: "It's not about me; it's about the hope that we can stay clean one day at a time." His remarks concluded with a metaphor on present-centered self-acceptance: "Dance like no one is watching!"

As we were leaving, I found Billy's wife (whom I first met along with Billy at my fellowship's annual statewide convention in Arizona a few months earlier) and told her how honored I was to be there. She turned to me, and with the kind of eye contact that momentarily stops time, replied, "We're honored to have you here." This touched my heart in a way that has no words, and I knew with every molecule of my being that she genuinely meant it, yet it was difficult for me to believe. I was blessed just to be there, why would anyone be "honored" by my presence? Slowly but progressively, I've begun to understand how such a thing is possible.

The twelve-step gestalt reinforces that when we share our pain, it is lessened, and when we share our joy, it becomes greater. When I am the recipient of compassion in response to baring my soul, it nurtures my capacity to be more compassionate toward others, and toward myself. We can identify and empathize with each other's experience because we have all been there and done that. The details may differ, but the process, the feelings, and many of the patterns of thinking are universal, binding us together through the tribulations of shared experience. Even if we have never met previously, we know each other.

It was also during my first year in recovery that my father turned eighty, and chose to celebrate this momentous birthday on the beach in southern Delaware, where my daughters and I, along with my brother and sisters and their families, would share two adjoining townhouses for a week. I hadn't seen my entire family of origin in several years, and this was going to be my first visit with them since I went to treatment. From the time I moved from Long Island to LA at the age of seventeen, I had spent every visit with my parents and siblings under the influence of whatever I could put my hands on, from the time I got up in the morning until I went to sleep at night. Using provided a way to steel myself to the deluge of energy and mixed emotions that flowed from our collective presence, the remnants of the past swirling around us whenever we gathered together. No one knows how to push each other's buttons—whether intentionally or unconsciously—quite like immediate family.

Looking at traveling 2,100 miles to a place I had never been before for an extended visit in close quarters with nineteen family members without the use of drugs set off alarm bells in my head. I shared about my anxiety with Phil and at meetings. After one such meeting, my friend Michael, who then had fourteen years in recovery, told me that prior to moving to Tucson he lived in Bethany Beach, Delaware—the same small town where my family was staying. What are the chances of that? He gave me the location and lowdown on three different meetings in that area. Michael then gave me the name and phone number of his sponsor who still lived there, and said he would call Terry to let him know that I was coming into town and that I would be contacting him. How the hell does something like that happen?

My second evening in Bethany Beach, I met Terry at one of the meetings Michael recommended. I had never been to southern Delaware in my life, and obviously had never been to this meeting, yet as soon as it started, I felt at home. At the beginning of meetings, the chairperson will typically ask, "Is there anyone here from out of town?" When I responded, "Hi I'm Dan, and I'm an addict from Tucson, Arizona," I was warmly welcomed by the group. There were some small differences from the meetings I had become used to in Tucson, but my experience was much more the same than it was different. My twelve-step program gives me the experience of being able to feel at home, even in a place I've never been to before.

The next night Terry picked me up and took me to a different meeting. I understood why Michael wanted to keep him as a sponsor even though they now lived across the country from one another. Like Phil, he seemed the embodiment of recovery, imbued with unconditional acceptance and loving kindness, and freely giving of his time to someone he had never met before.

Throughout our time in Delaware, my parents and siblings were nothing but respectful and supportive of the needs of my recovery. I think they were holding their collective breath a little, not knowing what to expect or how I would be. They literally hadn't experienced me abstinent from mind- and mood-altering substances for more than a few hours at a time since I was sixteen. Though not lacking in emotional intensity, the visit overall was extremely positive, allowing us to reconnect and celebrate my father's birthday in a spirit of family and love that we all deserved.

While there is no such thing as a perfect support system, my particular twelve-step program may come as close to it as is humanly possible. Anything that involves people is subject to the full range of human frailties, and my twelve-step program is no exception. However, it is guided by commitment to a clear and unwavering common purpose, functioning as a rudder that steers the program and those who participate in it actively in the direction of growth and healing.

It is a support system with twenty-four/seven availability—depending on geographic area, there are meetings available every day, throughout the year, often from morning until night. On certain major holidays such as Thanksgiving, Christmas, and New Year's Eve many communities schedule special activities, including "marathon meetings" that run continuously throughout the day. These events are planned to help those in recovery cope with the stresses and strong emotions often created by the holidays. There are online meetings and chat rooms for those in more rural areas with fewer in-person meetings. Program members reach out to those who are new, giving to others that which was given to them—simultaneously giving back to the fellowship while paying forward the message that recovery is possible and support is available.

My twelve-step program provides access to multiple levels of support that I think of as concentric circles, including one's sponsor, who functions as a guide and mentor; close friends in recovery, who comprise a more individualized support group; one's home group—the meeting that provides a consistent anchor for meeting attendance; other fellowship members, and meetings locally, statewide, nationally, and internationally. Mine is a global support system—a truly worldwide, multilingual, multicultural fellowship with more than 58,000 weekly meetings in 131 countries.

As a result of my professional life in behavioral health, I've spent time on both sides of the desk in therapy. It is generally strongly recommended that anyone who provides therapy to others have the experience of being in therapy themselves. When I was thirty-one, I was in therapy with Bob, the brilliant psycho-dynamically oriented clinical psychologist who interpreted my calling my mother by her first name starting in seventh grade. For all of his knowledge and expertise, Bob did not have experience in treating addiction—though of course that wasn't why I was seeing him.

At the time, I was the Clinical Director of Network, the residential substance abuse treatment program for adolescents in Rockleigh, NJ. My position was part of the civil service system in Bergen County, which provided by far the most generous mental health benefits I've ever had. My motivation at the time was to use this opportunity for personal growth and professional development.

During one of our sessions, I described in detail my history of drug use (which wouldn't be concluded for another seventeen years). Bob looked at me intently and said, "I'm surprised, I would never have expected that from what I know of you." A familiar feeling of being judged with its attendant shame started to rise, when he stated very simply, "You must have been in a lot of pain." I began to tear up, but quickly suppressed it, putting the reaction back in the box where I kept my emotions of vulnerability contained. I wasn't yet capable of permitting the pain he had touched and the sadness that started to emerge and threatened to overwhelm me, its natural expression. But, in that moment, I felt more deeply understood than I ever had in my entire life—until I came to the rooms of twelve-step recovery.

chapter twelve

[WOULD YOU RATHER BE RIGHT OR] WOULD YOU RATHER BE HAPPY?

"When I let go of what I am,
I become what I might be."

LAO TZU

A striking and paradoxical feature shared by many people struggling with addiction is sometimes described in twelve-step recovery as "being an egomaniac with an inferiority complex." Internally, deep down, we feel inadequate, damaged, broken, "not good enough" (or simply "not enough") or "less than." These feelings and the beliefs they are based on usually have their origins in the messages received from others starting early in life. How we react in the present is strongly influenced by childhood experiences and internalized beliefs.

The wreckage that active addiction leaves in its wake serves to reinforce and deepen the self-perception that there is something fundamentally wrong with us. As I've described, these beliefs and the resultant feelings are often so distressing that addicts protect themselves by keeping them unconscious. Occasionally, there may be some awareness of their existence, but due to the discomfort they create they tend to remain hidden—from oneself, as well as from everyone else. They also affect (or perhaps infect) most all ongoing relationships.

One way in which beliefs and feelings of inferiority can be disguised or kept at a distance is through the defense mechanism of reaction-formation. Reaction-formation protects against painful thoughts and feelings by turning them into their opposites—for example, presenting an attitude of arrogance—that I'm not "less than" others because I am "better than" others! However, this form of self-protection takes considerable energy to maintain since it constantly requires having to demonstrate that superiority to everyone, including oneself. This often manifests in the need to be in control, the need to "be right," and effectively lifting oneself up by putting others down. This occurs whenever I judge people in a negative way—I am implicitly putting them down, making them inferior, and elevating the way I see myself by making myself "superior" to them.

A common feature of such an attitude of superiority is believing and acting as if one knows what's best regardless of the situation. Prior to recovery, it was standard procedure for me to try to control people and situations based on what I thought was best, and the need to be right convinced me of the correctness of my approach. The need to be right involves being intolerant of and rejecting others' viewpoints. When someone is emotionally attached to the need to be right, when the ideas or suggestions of others differ from his or hers, then those other perspectives must be "wrong."

The further I sank into the tar pit of my active addiction and chronic pain during the final couple of years before getting clean, the greater my need for control became. As my life became increasingly unmanageable and out of control, I compensated by becoming more controlling—of situations and other people—another excellent example of reaction-formation in action. These attempts to control took both overt and indirect forms as I argued, demanded, asserted, manipulated, steered, suggested, cajoled, pleaded, played on sympathy (especially sympathy engendered by my pain), and generally did whatever it took to get the outcome I wanted—and on some level, believed that I had to have.

Obviously, a need for control and to be "right" is not unique to those of us challenged with addiction (though it is one of our specialties). In my family of origin, my father is legendary for his controlling behaviors, which seem to emanate from an insistent need to be right. Because he is brilliant and extremely well-versed in a wide array of subjects, frequently he is, in fact, right. However, even when talking to someone with much more experience and knowledge in a given area, he is impressively steadfast in trying to impose his view.

This need to be right often had the feel of intellectual or emotional bullying that could be obnoxious to the point of being painful to be around. It could also alienate people. In the fall of 2010, I watched my father argue about Western medicine and the Canadian medical system with Ralph. Ralph is a retired physician and former Joint Commission on Accreditation of Health Care Organizations (now known as The Joint Commission) surveyor who attended medical school and practiced medicine in Canada, prior to moving to the US where he also practiced for decades. Ralph had extensive experience and real expertise in the healthcare systems of both countries, and therefore could possibly know just a little more about this topic than my father. As he started to rev-up, I reminded him of Ralph's background and qualifications, but did that dissuade him from pressing forward with his disagreements? Hell, it didn't even slow him down. I wanted to grab him and say, "Please . . . just fucking stop already!"

In child and human development there is a natural tendency to become like our most important role models, particularly our same-sex primary parent figures. In other words, boys tend to take on characteristics of their father figures and girls those of their mother figures. The main processes through which this phenomenon takes place are identification and social learning. Identification is a psychological process whereby people take on aspects, qualities, or attributes of another, and effectively become more like that other person. Some people take on only a few of the qualities of the parent figure while others may become very much like them, i.e., "He's just like his father." "You're exactly like your mother!" Like many of the psychological processes I've described, identification occurs outside of our conscious awareness. This is apparent when people make a deliberate commitment that they "will never be like my father" (or mother), and yet over time, they still end up taking on some of the very characteristics they may have despised in their parent figures.

Social learning occurs when people learn new information and behaviors by observing other people—most often important role models—and how they act and react in various situations, as well as what happens as a result of their actions. Here again, our most influential role models growing up tend to be our same sex primary parent figures. Whatever attitudes, beliefs, and behaviors we observe in our same sex parent figures, we are more likely to imitate, taking on those behaviors ourselves. Another level of social learning takes place through our interactions with others. Behaviors that are positively reinforced by getting desired results—what we want consciously or unconsciously (for instance, being in control or being "right") are apt to be repeated.

I became progressively more controlling toward my wife and daughters, driven by

- my burgeoning sense of unmanageability as my active addiction and chronic pain progressed;

- the increasing levels of pain, anxiety, fear, inadequacy, loss, and self-loathing it engendered;

- my need to compensate for feeling out-of-control;

- some identification with my father; and,

- the influences of social learning.

I tried to direct my wife and daughters as if our day-to-day lives were a major motion picture. Increasingly, I needed to be right, and generally *knew* that I was. And if they would simply listen to me and do the things I wanted them to do the way I wanted them done—because I was right, dammit—then everything would be fine.

I dictated such things as how suitcases needed to be packed in preparation for family trips—not just my suitcase, but everyone's. After all, I had been taught the art and science of using all available packing space to maximum efficiency by my mother, who had been taught by my grandmother. My thinking assured me that the efficient use of limited available space—for items in each suitcase, for each suitcase in the car, etc.—required my direct oversight. It would get to the point where I would inspect their suitcases to ensure that each one was packed well enough. If it wasn't, I had to repack it myself (taking total control) or engage in a wrestling match inside my head—the intellectual understanding that the most helpful and healthy thing I could do would be to back off and allow them the space to do it their own way vs. my obsessive-compulsive need for control.

This dynamic was never more evident than when I did interior painting in our various homes, first in New York, and then in Arizona. Although it plays to stereotype, in my experience the list of great Jewish handymen is a short one, and rarely did I observe my father wielding a hammer, screwdriver, or home repair/improvement tools of any sort. I had little personal frame of reference for do-it-yourself handiwork until my Italian Catholic father in-law showed me how to do a few things. He had worked in construction most of his adult life, and was partially disabled because of a six-foot fall from a scaffold in his early sixties.

He taught me the fundamentals of quality interior painting, and I put that learning to considerable use, painting much of the interiors of three different homes. Never having been artistic in traditional ways, I enjoyed the artistry of using colors that correlated with and complemented one another and adding "designer" touches such as customized borders around windows, ceilings, and floors. Moreover, interior painting made for a complete contrast with my work in behavioral health. By virtue of the complexity of counseling, involving as it does so many different variables, clear successes are all too few and often fleeting. Positive outcomes are frequently tinged with ambiguity, and their durability is always uncertain. With interior painting, the "before" and "after" differences are dramatic, and the results are unmistakable and enduring.

I was meticulous in every aspect of the process, often spending as much or more time on the prep work as I did on the actual painting. Everything about the job at hand was systematic and precise. I didn't just put drop cloths down; I folded each one to shape, placing it carefully, prior to using masking tape to keep them in place and minimize the chances of paint getting on the floor. My use of specialized painting tape to define edges and shapes was painstakingly detail-oriented. And the paint itself had to be applied correctly and with great care, using the proper tools for each aspect of the job—edgers, rollers of different dimensions, and brushes in a range of sizes. The objective was always to have immaculate, straight lines and leave no visible drips or other inconsistencies. In other words, it had to be perfect, or damn near as close as a human being could get to it.

It was a scenario tailor-made for my perfectionism: not only could I act on it without creating (much) upset for myself or others, but it was an adaptive, helping me to achieve the result I sought and adding beauty to the aesthetic of our homes. Left to my own devices, I could control the shit out of it, agonizing about the process and obsessing over its outcome as much as I felt the need to. And it worked really well, until my darling daughters wanted to help.

They wanted to help as kids do naturally, especially when these projects involved painting their rooms. Painting their rooms to their specifications was a special gift that I adored giving to them. They were given wide latitude to select the colors and designs they wanted, and I would make it happen. All they wanted was to participate, to do this together with me, and to experience the accomplishment of contributing. This occurred with both of my daughters, at different times, on several occasions when they were between the ages of about six and fourteen. I would have loved to have been able to let them help me. It would have been a beautiful experience to share with them.

However, I just couldn't fucking do it. Every time I attempted to paint with them I quickly devolved into an impatient, intolerant asshole. They would do the best they could, but it wasn't good enough for me. Their brush strokes were off; there were drips and other imperfections where they painted; and they would make minor messes here and there. And internally, it drove me crazy. I so wanted to do this with them, as well as for them. They were doing as well as they were capable of, but I was incapable of appreciating and accepting that. I was never able to allow them to help me paint for very long, and this inability created suffering for everyone involved.

It was a lose-lose scenario; even when I eased off and made a conscious effort to relinquish some control, I had nonverbal ways of making clear that I wasn't happy about their performance. A disapproving glance or an exasperated tone of voice expressed my dissatisfaction and sent the message that in that moment, they were not good enough.

I have vivid recollections of being on the receiving end of those glances and that tone. I learned first-hand how hurtful they can be and the staying power that hurt can have. I knew all too well that these kinds of experiences damage the developing sense of self—they cut like a jagged piece of glass, bleeding off self-worth. Every such glance and utterance is an act of subtle (and sometimes not-so-subtle) emotional rejection and abandonment, a psychological betrayal of parent to child. Each of these episodes became another brick in the wall separating me emotionally from my family. The more I was unable to control my own actions, the more invested I became in controlling theirs. In my need to be right, I was horribly wrong.

Typically, within seconds of perpetrating these hurts, I recoiled in guilt and shame. Guilt at my behavior—how, especially as a trained therapist, I *knew* better, and knew my kids deserved better; and shame at my deficiency as a parent and how I should *be* better. I had conducted many therapy sessions specific to parenting, designed and administered parent education programs and parenting groups, and facilitated numerous staff trainings related to parenting and family systems issues. And yet, the need to bind my escalating anxiety and fear by attaching them to something concrete and outside of myself compelled me to repeat this behavior in one form or another, over and over and over.

Each time I acted like this, I hated myself. Knowing I was wrong and wanting to both take responsibility and try to make reparations, I would apologize to my daughters, time after time. It got old for all of us. After you apologize for something, for anything, often enough, it becomes a rote exercise devoid of real meaning. When I close my eyes, I can still see the hurt etched on my daughters' faces.

The more unmanageable my life became, the more desperately I held on to the need to be "right." The past has a way of flooding the present, but it doesn't have to. While in treatment in Las Vegas, I was talking with a member of the medical staff in the chronic pain program about being in conflict with my wife. I shared with him my frustration that we were unable to come to anything approximating a meeting of minds in a specific situation where I "knew" that I was right. He told me the story of an ongoing argument he had been having with his own wife. The actual subject of such an argument could be virtually anything, and is much less important than the process. On the issue at hand, he and his wife strongly disagreed, each convinced that they were right. They both stubbornly held their ground, refusing to budge or back down. The only thing they could agree on in this matter was to seek the counsel of their pastor.

The husband knew that the pastor would side with his position, designating him as "right." As they shared their dramatically different perspectives, the husband made mental preparations to declare victory. To his considerable surprise, the pastor didn't take sides at all, gracefully sidestepping the dichotomy of right/wrong, and the zero sum game that went with it. Rather, he asked matter-of-factly, "Do you want to be right or do you want to be happy?"

I was stunned by the elegant simplicity and remarkable depth of that question. It instantly struck a chord that resonated in my heart, unlocking the door to an awareness that this could be a conscious choice. Until that very moment, I had been asleep to that possibility. My need to be right, and by extension my need to control people, situations, and outcomes has often obstructed my ability to be happy, insofar as happiness is a function of contentment and peace of mind, otherwise known as serenity. My need to be "right" and in control also made it difficult, if not impossible, for those closest to me to be happy or at peace.

As the *Tao Te Ching* describes in verse 74:

> Trying to control things
>
> is like trying to take the master carpenter's place.
>
> When you handle the master carpenter's tools,
>
> chances are that you'll cut yourself.

And then blood gets all over the place and it's a big fucking mess!

Do I want to be right or do I want to be happy? Which is more important? Which is healthier? Which is more recovery supportive? Which promotes my alignment with a spiritual connection to that which is greater than myself? Which brings me closer to those I love, and closer to the person I'm meant to be—my true self? Looking at the two options through this lens makes the choice very simple.

In the years since, I've heard this choice reinforced in the rooms of twelve-step recovery. Whenever I can take a step back from the intensity of the circumstance and consciously consider the question, it's a slam dunk. Relinquishing the need to be right creates the space that makes it possible for me to experience greater happiness, contentment, and peace of mind. This revelation is only reaffirmed as the days, weeks, months, and years roll by and time becomes more precious.

Successful, sustained recovery requires two levels of change: awareness and action. Without awareness, the ability to take necessary action is limited. And yet, as essential as awareness is, by itself it is of limited value. During the early to mid-twentieth century, it was not uncommon to treat addiction exclusively with psychoanalysis or other forms of psychotherapy. This approach was based on the view that addiction was the result of unresolved and unconscious conflicts, often stemming from childhood experiences. These efforts helped to create a group of addicts who demonstrated excellent insight as to why they used alcohol and other drugs to excess, but their active addiction and all of its serious concomitant problems continued unabated.

We might like to believe that if we know our behavior is problematic and unhealthy, and if we can identify the underlying motivations for this "bad" behavior, we'll stop doing it. In reality, not so much. It is entirely possible to understand the reasons why we engage in self-defeating behaviors that generate all sorts of adverse consequences and still continue to do the exact same things. All of my professional knowledge and awareness didn't keep me from doing the same things that repeatedly created suffering for me and those closest to me. I kept banging my head against those same walls over and over and over again. And, the only positive experience I've ever had related to banging my head against any wall is how good it feels when I finally stop.

One of the ways I've worked to apply this recovery-oriented awareness and stop banging my head against a very familiar wall is in my interactions with my father. When we reach an impasse where it's clear that we can't find common ground and any constructive meeting of our minds is unlikely, I've learned to simply say something along the lines of "Dad, it's not going to be helpful for us to talk about this (whatever it is) any further for now. Clearly, we're not going to be able to agree on it, and we're going to have to agree to disagree, because continuing to discuss it now will serve no useful purpose, and nothing positive will come of it."

The first five or six times I used this approach, it was as if I hadn't said anything at all. He didn't acknowledge it and kept right on talking, repeating his perspective and attempting to convince me of its correctness. My challenge lay in being conscious of my emotional reactions including my own need to be right, keep them separate from my behavior, and remain centered and focused. Whenever I've been able to do this while reiterating the above statements in a matter-of-fact way, after several repetitions, to his credit my father has been able to hear them and respond positively. We are then freed to change topics and continue our interaction (whether by phone or in person) without getting mired in escalating conflict and negativity. When it happens, this is a great gift that we have given to ourselves, to each other, and to our relationship. In effect, we've exchanged the need to be right for greater contentment and serenity—at least for that moment.

In my interactions with my daughters, I make a concerted and conscious effort to remain aware of my reactions and give them the space to say what they need to say and do what they need to do, without attempting to direct or control the situation. My younger daughter was a sophomore at Northern Arizona University in Flagstaff, Arizona, when she took the bus to Las Vegas (where I have been living since 2008) to spend Thanksgiving with me. It was shortly after I celebrated five years in recovery, and I was excited and grateful for the opportunity to have an extended visit with just the two of us. I spent considerable time and energy planning our menu, conferring with her to ensure it included whatever she wanted to eat. I wanted everything to go as well as it possibly could and became attached to that outcome.

On Thanksgiving morning I was obsessing about the preparation and timing of the main meal, when my daughter arose and I had to shift my attention to breakfast. We agreed that she would make the eggs mixed with veggies while I continued to focus on the turkey and trimmings. She had been living in an off-campus apartment with three roommates for several months and was gaining experience in basic cooking. As she mixed the ingredients and started to cook, I realized that she wasn't doing it "right."

She was going to throw the raw onions in with the eggs without cooking them down first! Having to intervene, I convinced her to cook the onions separately prior to adding them—*whew*. Then to my horror, not only did she select the "wrong" type of pan, but she also put the egg mixture into the pan before oiling it. She assured me that this was how she did it at home and it worked fine, but I was unmoved. With the stress level in the room rising, I began to launch into a lecture about proper food preparation and cooking technique when I caught myself.

I was trying to control even the small details of her participation in what was supposed to be a shared effort. Here we were, father and daughter working together cooperatively in what was a beautiful moment, and my need to be right was on the verge of fucking it up. In stark contrast to what I would have done before I found recovery, I took a deep breath and a big-ass step back. I told her that she could make the eggs whatever way she thought was best, and that I was sure they would turn out well. And I knew in that moment, the eggs would be fine. The joy of our experience together would lay in our process rather than any specific culinary outcome. Liberated from the bondage of my self-serving perspective, I was able to honor my daughter's desire to contribute and get the hell out of the way. We had a Thanksgiving with much to be grateful for and a great visit.

This is a perpetual work in progress for me. The more I can accept where my daughters are, the more they can experience feeling accepted by me without conditions. This is one of the keys to self-acceptance, and it is one of the gifts they deserve and that I need to give them. I don't have to agree with or like everything they do in order to accept them unconditionally. The more I can let go of my impulse to be right, the more opportunities I give to them and me to be content and even happy.

As I noted earlier, awareness does not by itself change behavior; the only way to change behavior is to do things differently. While awareness is a critical component of this process, translating awareness to action can be a significant challenge. It requires disengaging from the incessant internal dialogue and the unconscious autopilot mode that directs me to continue doing what I've become so used to doing. This involves conscious, ongoing reminders to self and takes no small amount of dedicated effort. I have to practice applying specific principles and using the tools of recovery daily and throughout each day. It doesn't matter how much oxygen I breathed yesterday; if I don't make sure to breathe today I'm in serious trouble. Further, I have to practice applying the skills I've learned, not just in the abstract, or when things are going smoothly, but especially when I'm under the influence of strong emotion(s) or circumstances of serious stress—when some sort of shit is hitting the fan.

chapter thirteen

[FROM AWARENESS TO ACTION]

"Which ever way your pleasure tends
If you plant ice you're gonna harvest wind."
ROBERT HUNTER, *FRANKLIN'S TOWER*, GRATEFUL DEAD

In order to be successful in and sustain recovery—or any process of meaningful change—both awareness *and* action are requisite. Translating conscious awareness into intentional action in recovery is similar to the process of learning and developing new skills in sports or other pursuits that necessitate performance in the face of varying degrees of stress or pressure.

At first glance, the following material might seem totally unrelated to recovery. However, the intimate interconnections of life find ways to tie all aspects of our experience together, no matter how disparate they may seem initially. Since they are often challenging to find, it can be easy to believe that these linkages between very different facets of our lives don't exist. Sometimes I have to look harder, look through a different lens, or look in a different place, but by looking carefully, with enough resourcefulness and creativity, I invariably find those connections. They are always there, patiently awaiting my discovery.

When I was fourteen I made a commitment to myself to learn a specific new basketball shot—a left-handed double-pump reverse layup. I was determined to make this shot part of my repertoire and master it to the best of my ability. Although I didn't consciously consider the various ingredients of the learning process at the time, it turned out that building this skill so I could use it effectively under pressure in competition involved several levels of awareness and application.

My primary motivations at the time were two-fold: it's a very creative and sophisticated shot that I knew would be an excellent skill-development challenge (in part because I'm right-handed), and in competition it yields the practical and strategic advantage of being unexpected and difficult to defend—it would give my game an additional and potent option. Truth be told, it's also an especially cool-looking move that often impresses observers and opponents alike—whenever I could score *and* look cool in action, it was the best of both worlds!

Like many recovery-related skills, meditation for example, this shot actually consists of several component parts, each of which needed to be developed and refined, before I could assemble the pieces together to form the entire sequence of actions. It begins with an aggressive dribble drive to the right side of the basket. Normally the defense assumes that if the person driving to the basket is going to shoot, it will happen here— on the right side, especially if that person is right-handed.

The shot then involves

- continuing the dribble drive underneath the basket;

- jumping to become airborne while still underneath the basket;

- switching the ball from the right hand to the left hand;

- double-pumping in order to stay in the air as forward momentum carries the body to the left side of the basket; and

- finishing with a left-handed mini-hook shot (to maximize the distance between the release of the ball and any defenders trying to block the shot) off the backboard using varying degrees of spin, depending upon the precise positioning of the body relative to the rim: the further underneath the rim, the more spin is necessary to get the ball from where it hits the backboard into the basket.

It's a complicated shot (even describing it in detail is complicated), and the entire sequence needs to happen at high speed to maximize its effectiveness.

At first, I practiced the individual elements separately. Then I practiced the entire sequence by myself at half speed or slower. When I had established a good-enough foundation to make this new shot with some consistency, I began to practice it by myself at full-speed. Subsequently, I started to use it in pick-up games and at team practices against defenders attempting to guard me and stop me from scoring. Ultimately, I was able to apply it in the heat of the most intense live competition—in actual games where I was accountable to my coach and my teammates, as well as to my own expectations.

It took literally thousands of practice runs and live applications of my left-handed double-pump reverse layup, under a wide range of conditions— on outdoor courts with different surfaces in a range of weather conditions, in addition to the hardwood indoors, and with diverse levels of competition—to master this complex, high-degree-of-difficulty shot.

The real test of one's learning and ability to apply that learning *in any area* is what happens when we perform under stress—when we are being challenged in some way. It's easy to be successful when there is no competition, or the competition is weak and the opposing team is lousy. When the opposition is tough and the full-court press is on, it's a sea change; uncertainty arises, and fear creeps into awareness. Self-doubt and confusion created by a swirling undercurrent of uncomfortable emotion take an adverse toll on performance in any area, and with surprising suddenness, momentum can shift and success that seemed secure becomes questionable.

This is especially true for recovery. It can seem impressively easy when life is going smoothly and all seems well. It's not unusual for people, particularly in the earlier phases of recovery (once the storm of post-acute withdrawal has passed), to be lulled into the false belief that it will always be so. However, as it's said in the rooms of twelve-step recovery, "life has a way of showing up." The real test of a person's recovery is how they respond when presented with serious challenges—in relationships, health, finances, job/career, etc. When the shit hits the fan (and sooner or later it always does, for everyone), my ability to be successful depends on how well I have developed the skills of recovery through dedicated learning and consistent practice. This is the essence of translating awareness into action.

The process of changing patterns of living requires conscious (a.k.a. mindful) and conscientious awareness, along with extraordinary patience and persistent practice. This applies to moving from a life in active addiction and chronic pain to one in recovery from both. It also ties in to my evolution (still very much a work in progress) from the need to be right to remaining mindful of and practicing the value of being content and at peace.

The most effective way to acquire new skills in any area—be it sports, reading, cooking, auto repair, using a computer, gardening, plumbing, meditating, or recovery—is to learn what works and practice what works with consistency and persistence.

Although I started smoking pot at the age of twelve, it wasn't until I was a freshman in college that I learned to roll a decent joint. I had a ton of expertise in the ins-and-outs of using pipes, my bong technique was flawless; a model of breath control and timing, and I had smoked hundreds of joints—but I couldn't roll one worth a damn. I just assumed that joint rolling was intuitive and either people knew how to do it or they didn't, and I didn't.

At the beginning of my freshman year at UC Santa Cruz, I met Andy. He came from the Kona coast on the big island of Hawaii and could roll a perfect joint the size of his thumb. We lived in the same dorm, and fueled by certain common interests, quickly became friends. Andy would use a single tiny, rice paper-thin rolling paper to produce a work of functional art, a massive yet perfect cylinder that burned flawlessly.

I was in awe, and figured that if anyone could help me learn how to roll a proper doobie, it was Andy. Even if I could never approximate the artistry or scale of his work, under Andy's tutelage, I learned the three techniques essential to joint rolling. Having learned the techniques that worked, I had to practice them rigorously in order to develop the level of skill I sought—and I did.

I went through the same process when I committed to learning how to eat with chopsticks, also shortly after arriving at UC Santa Cruz. Prior to that, I had attempted to use chopsticks only once and failed thoroughly. I made the conscious decision that I was going to become competent in using them, regardless of how foolish I looked or inept I felt during the learning process. Someone with considerably greater experience and skill than me taught the essential techniques, and then I practiced the shit out of them. It took about four months before I developed the level of skill I sought.

Progress is rarely a straight line. It can be slow and halting. Typically it's two steps forward and one step back; sometimes it feels like one step forward and two steps back. But, if I stay this course, gradually and progressively, my performance in any area improves.

The process of learning and skill development has four stages according to Milton Erickson, MD, a psychiatrist and psychotherapist who had an extraordinary grasp of human perception, information processing, and behavior, with an emphasis on unconscious processes. His revolutionary work in clinical hypnosis was so far ahead of its time that it essentially brought that method into the twenty-first century—even though Erickson himself passed away in 1980. His innovative theories and artful approaches to helping people influenced the development of brief psychotherapy, strategic family therapy, and family systems therapy, and contributed directly to the genesis of solution-focused therapy and Neuro-Linguistic Programming (NLP).

Erickson's four stages of learning—unconscious incompetence, conscious incompetence, conscious competence, and unconscious competence—characterize virtually any skill development process. For instance, people who learn how to read well and who develop mastery in reading, progress through each of these stages. And although I was unaware of it at the time, they were evident in the development of my left-handed double-pump reverse layup in early adolescence.

Unconscious incompetence is a state of obliviousness—not knowing something, but also not knowing that we don't know it and therefore, not caring about it one way or another. Before I started thinking about the idea of developing a left-handed double-pump reverse layup, I was unconsciously incompetent with regard to it. I didn't even know that I did not know how to make this shot.

At the point that I determined I wanted to learn the left-handed double-pump reverse layup and make it part of my hoops arsenal, I progressed to conscious incompetence. In other words, I became consciously aware of the shot and its potential value, and knew that I did not yet have the skill and experience to use it proficiently. In terms of this shot, I was functionally incompetent.

Gradually, as the result of rigorous ongoing practice, testing and fine-tuning the component parts of the shot and putting them together into a coherent whole, I was able to achieve conscious competence. I became very good at making the shot in varying conditions; however, when performing this complex move I had to think intentionally about each aspect of it—the speed and rhythm of my dribble drive on the approach to the basket, the positioning of my body relative to the defender guarding me, the timing of my jump, the positioning of my body relative to the basket, the timing of the release of the ball, as well as the distance to the rim and how much spin to put on the ball to bank it off the backboard and into the basket.

It was only through careful and conscious application of my left-handed double-pump reverse layup during many hundreds of hours of practice and live competition, that my ability to use it reached the level of unconscious competence. At that point, I no longer had to think about how to perform this complex shot. The various parts had merged seamlessly into a single continuum that began with the dribble drive down the right side of the court toward the basket and concluded with the ball banking off the backboard on the left side and going through the rim and into the net. Through countless repetitions I had learned it so well that I could do it automatically.

Unconscious competence is also known as mastery. When athletes are described as being "in the zone," they are in a state of unconscious competence. They are performing at such a high level that they seem unstoppable. Yet, every aspect of their performance may appear effortless, almost as if they were operating on autopilot. It is as if they are in sync with the universe and have tapped into its cadence.

Basketball is an excellent metaphor for recovery. On the court, as in real life, the environment and its circumstances evolve continuously. The action is constant, but energy and momentum can shift dramatically. Different players rotate in and out of the game, some playing more substantial roles than others. Each person's playing time and the significance of his or her role can change. Coaches and assistant coaches are resources that help to provide direction, guidance, and mentoring. Even the best players require the support of teammates in order to win games. And even the best teams have to call time-out on occasion, when the game gets away from them, and they need to regroup.

In order to be successful, it's important to be able to see as much of the court as possible, to be present-centered and mindfully aware of what's happening in the moment. What is the overall defense doing? Is it a full-court press, a half-court trap, a man-to-man, or a zone? Is the defense laying back to prevent the dribble drive and giving up the outside shot? Or it is playing close and tight, creating opportunities to drive to the hoop? Success against each type of defense requires a different set of responses. Successfully negotiating life on its own terms requires a similar assessment of the situations I am presented with in the here and now.

The more present-centered and mindful I am, the more intentionally I can act; the more choices I have—in basketball or any other area of life, including recovery. Conversely, the more stressed, pressured, or anxious I feel the more impulsive and reactive I'm likely going to be, and the more likely I am to make unnecessary mistakes. The more different options, skills, and tools I have, the better prepared I am to successfully cope with changing situations and whatever comes next. Continuing the basketball metaphor, this means being able to handle the ball with both right and left hands; being able to drive to the rack and shoot effectively with either hand from close range; being able to make a high percentage of my free throws; having a consistent outside shot that extends to three-point range; and having a variety of low post moves, including a jump hook and classic hook shot, along with a fade-away turnaround jumper going right or left.

John Wooden was the legendary men's basketball coach at UCLA whose teams achieved an unparalleled degree of success. They won ten national championships during a twelve year span from 1963 to 1975. Wooden thought of himself first and foremost as an educator; a teacher whose primary responsibility was to prepare the young men he coached to be successful in life, rather than just in basketball. He did this by teaching and instilling in his players an incredible foundation of values in addition to skills, through continuous repetition.

It's unclear if Coach Wooden knew of Milton Erickson's model for learning and skill development. What is clear is that he was intimately familiar with the concept of unconscious competence/mastery and sought to operationalize it at the team level. His approach to preparing his teams was based on uncompromising conditioning and meticulous execution achieved through the mastery of universal team and individual fundamentals. His teams achieved a degree of unconscious competence by practicing virtually the same way every time they took the court. Coach Wooden taught that failing to prepare translated into preparing to fail. He maintained an unwavering belief that if his teams practiced the right things the right way and performed to the best of their ability, winning would take care of itself; and it did.

As challenging as it can be to learn and develop new skills in any area, in comparison to recovery all the examples I've described are simple and concrete. Skills such as accepting things I really, really want to change, but can't, and tolerating distressing emotions and physical sensations without acting on them in ways that make situations worse are incredibly difficult to master. At least to this point, in recovery I am very rarely unconsciously competent. Moreover, skillful recovery requires a high degree of moment-to-moment conscious attention and awareness. To acquire this level of conscious awareness to the point where it becomes second nature suggests a level of spiritual development that may well be beyond the reach of all but the most enlightened among us. While achieving anything but occasional unconscious competence in recovery may not be realistic for most of us, becoming increasingly consciously competent and skillful in recovery from both addiction and chronic pain surely is.

When it comes to developing recovery-supporting skills and effectively bringing them to bear, especially in the heat of the moment, conscious competence is challenging enough to achieve and maintain. It is only through the ongoing practice of applying conscious awareness and the consistent repetition of recovery-supporting actions that I give myself the opportunity to continue my progress.

Riding a bike, reading, playing catch, keyboarding/typing, and playing video games are examples of everyday activities that progress through Erickson's four stages of learning—improving with practice and repetition to become unconscious and automatic. Once a skill has been learned well enough to be successfully applied in action, it becomes an available resource that can not only be applied in a range of circumstances, but also expanded. In other words, once somebody has learned how to read it doesn't matter whether the length of a book is ten pages or three-hundred pages; once you know how to swim, you can swim in water that's four feet deep or four hundred feet deep. The same dynamic applies to recovery-oriented skills.

And yet, mastery is a fluid rather than a static entity. Like recovery itself, it is an ongoing journey rather than a particular destination. Whenever I discontinue doing the things I've learned to do that contribute to the unconscious competence I've experienced in any area of life, then that mastery always deteriorates. And when it does, I invariably find myself regressing to lower levels of skill. Activities I previously performed at high levels without thinking, again require conscious attention. It is a matter of using it or risk losing it.

The brain plays a central role in both active addiction and recovery. Brain imaging studies as reported by the US National Institute on Drug Abuse (NIDA) demonstrate that physical changes take place in areas of the brains of drug addicted individuals that affect learning, decision-making, judgment, memory, and behavior control. These brain changes can be long lasting, but most are neither permanent nor irreversible.

Until relatively recently, a prevailing scientific belief was that the structure of the human brain is set hard-and-fast in early childhood with all the neurons it will ever have. It was accepted as fact that no new neurons are added—ever, and that what is there is as good as it's ever going to get. According to this paradigm, the only possible changes in brain structure and functioning were negative—involving the loss of neurons and functioning due to traumatic injury, neurological illness, such as stroke or dementia, damage due to addiction, or the natural inevitable effects of aging.

It is now widely recognized that the brain has the ability to change and adapt throughout a person's life. This ability, known as neuroplasticity, allows the brain's structure and functioning to change in response to external stimuli, experience, and activity. Through the processes of thinking, learning, and acting, the brain continuously lays down new pathways for the processing and communicating of information and reorganizes existing ones.

The human brain adapts to repetitive experiences by forming memory connections or tracks. These connections are created by changes in brain structure and functioning, and work in the brain's operating system—outside of conscious awareness. When repeated consistently over time, any activity, behavior, or experience—whether healthy and positive or unhealthy and destructive—can create new unconscious memory tracks.

The formation of these memory tracks in the brain and body is what eventually allows activities to be performed without conscious thought or effort. This process is not unlike the grading and paving of a roadway that allows traffic to travel easily and efficiently. In the brain, over time the repetition of an activity can turn a dirt road into a freeway.

The brain changes both physically and functionally as connections between neurons are generated, rewired, and/or refined. It is the brain's capacity to make these changes that gives us the ability to memorize new facts, form new memories, adjust to new experiences and environments, integrate new learning, and develop new skills. The memory tracks that are created through repetitive experiences serve to deepen learning and strengthen mental, emotional, and muscle memory.

Habits, those patterns of behavior that develop through repetition, are the cause, as well as the result of these kinds of changes in the brain. Repetitive substance use creates new neural pathways and unconscious memory tracks. Similarly, because the nature of chronic pain is that it is an all-too repetitive experience, it also generates unconscious memory tracks.

The repetitive experiences and behaviors I engaged in over the course of the many years of my active addiction led to certain changes in my brain and created specific memory tracks. For example, my experience of pain— physical or emotional—translated instantly into a desire to use. These memory tracks became manifest in the literal habits of my addiction—the patterns, routines, and rituals that accompanied and reinforced thinking, feeling, and acting in ways that continued to fuel my using.

In recovery, my brain has had the opportunity to heal and rebuild the connections that were damaged and distorted during active addiction. Consistent with neuroplasticity, the brain is extremely resilient and has the ability to adapt to new and different repetitive experiences. That's what gives us older dogs the capacity to learn and master new tricks. Every day I have the opportunity to create memory pathways that support my recovery. By engaging in recovery-oriented experiences one day at a time these memory tracks form the foundation of my "habits" of recovery.

Since my addiction and chronic pain beat the crap out of me physically, mentally, emotionally, and spiritually, my approach to recovery for both needs to encompass these four domains. When I entered recovery, my skills in the domains of the mental and the physical were considerably more developed than in the latter two. However, my chronic pain condition had significantly depleted my physical abilities. I had dabbled in more focused spiritual pursuits on and off since the age of seventeen, and prior to going into treatment had been meditating on a nearly daily basis for the better part of ten years. And as a behavioral health professional with extensive training and experience in psychotherapy and clinical hypnosis, I had an excellent *theoretical* understanding of the emotional realm.

Where I was impoverished was in my ability to apply my knowledge of emotional and spiritual health and well-being in my own life—to translate my awareness into action. My efforts to do so were generally superficial and intellectualized at best. When under any sort of significant stress, as when the shit hit the fan in some way, I retreated into my head to try to understand, analyze, and make sense of it (whatever it was) and to help keep my emotions at a safe distance. To make certain that I numbed my emotions and changed the way I felt, I always got loaded. This was what I knew; and I rode that train until it ran out of track.

The heart of my habits of recovery from both addiction and chronic pain is an extensive daily morning practice that combines spiritual reading, meditation, nondenominational prayer, self-hypnosis, Egoscue stretching, and chi kung exercises. In microcosm, this daily practice integrates the physical, mental, emotional, and spiritual aspects of the recovery process. Like the left-handed double-pump reverse layup that I learned and mastered at the age of fourteen, it brings multiple elements together to form a more potent and meaningful whole.

Egoscue is a postural therapy method that treats chronic musculoskeletal pain using precise stretching exercises to bring the body back into proper alignment and restore function to muscles and joints. Chi kung, as I learned in treatment, is an ancient Chinese approach to health and healing that emphasizes the importance of aligning breath, physical activity, and conscious awareness. In blending gentle rhythmic movements, breathing techniques, and focused attention, chi kung helps to reduce stress, increase vitality, and enhance the immune system.

If translating awareness into action means learning the approaches and techniques that work, and then practicing them with persistence and dedication (and it does), consistency and repetition are key. Consistency and repetition are embedded in every aspect of my daily morning recovery practice. For starters, I do it like clockwork, rarely missing a day—and when I do miss a day, I can feel the difference. I do it in the early morning because that is the only time of day where I can consistently set aside the forty-five to fifty minutes it takes to complete, even though it requires me to get up much earlier than I would otherwise.

Each time I engage in this practice, I go through the same process, using the same structure (the same elements), sequence (the order of those elements), and amount of time spent (on the overall practice, as well as on each element). When at home, I use the same places in the same room. I have specific locations and body positions for each element, changing them only as I transition from one to the next. I do the spiritual reading and meditation seated on my bed, though I use slightly different postures for each; I move to the floor for the nondenominational prayer, self-hypnosis, and Egoscue stretching, and I go through the chi kung exercises while standing.

Through daily repetition, this multimodal recovery practice deepens the conscious and unconscious memory tracks that guide me further in the direction of health, healing, and wholeness. Neural pathways have been established that connect this practice with particular feeling states, memories, body positioning, and sensory stimuli. Consequently, for me, feelings of relaxation, calmness, and serenity have become directly associated with this practice and its component parts. Simply by assuming the same specific body position in the same location in the same room and beginning the first part of my daily morning practice, unconsciously and automatically my mind and body begin the process of becoming more calm, relaxed, and peaceful.

This recovery routine helps to enrich my spirit by strengthening my connection to that which is beyond me, and between the conscious and the unconscious parts of me, as well as between my outside and my inside. It shifts my attention from an orientation centered in my head to one centered in my heart and spirit, as each element of this practice creates a space that prompts me to translate my awareness of the healing value of nonjudgmental present-centered acceptance into action.

chapter fourteen

[BEING HERE NOW]

"Ripple in still water
When there is no pebble tossed
Nor wind to blow."
ROBERT HUNTER, *RIPPLE*, GRATEFUL DEAD

As twelve-step programs suggest, recovery happens "one day at a time." This slogan is a reminder that no one needs to spend time worrying about not using for the rest of his or her life. The idea of "never using again" tends to be so big that for many people it can be overwhelming. Those new to recovery can easily become discouraged, anxious, fearful, angry, or resentful when they think in terms of not using forever more. It's natural to think "There's no way I'm never going to use again . . . the rest of my life . . . it's just not possible!"

Believe it or not, thinking about not using for the rest of one's life is a waste of time and energy. Even if I'm committed to remaining abstinent for the duration of my time here on Earth, the reality is that I only need to focus on not using today. As it relates to using, even thinking about tomorrow makes little sense insofar as it is impossible to use tomorrow until it arrives. And when tomorrow arrives, it's now today.

Though it is not necessarily easy, especially for those new to recovery, not using "just for today" is realistic and entirely possible. The idea of it is much less intimidating and much more attainable. The most effective way to accomplish any huge goal or project is to break it down into smaller, more manageable parts. This is also a clinical technique known as partializing. By not using just for today, one day at a time, many people put together many years of recovery, and many never use again.

Recovery, and indeed life, occurs one day at a time. But really, they happen one moment at a time. Life unfolds in this very moment, right here and right now. And the vast majority of people are missing it. They are caught up in thinking about what happened in the past—a minute ago, an hour ago, yesterday, last week, two months ago, last year—or what may happen in the future—in a few minutes, an hour from now, tomorrow, next week, next month, etc. This is so common and so normal that often we don't even realize we're engaged in it. It happens automatically and unconsciously. (Note: this type of unconscious automatic state is the functional opposite of what occurs during the state of unconscious competence/mastery—the pinnacle of present-centeredness described in Chapter Twelve.)

Thoughts about what has happened or might happen pop into our heads and we run with them, often to cognitive and emotional places that have nothing whatsoever to do with this moment. We are somewhere other than here and now. This phenomenon occurs with such stunning regularity that for many, if not most people, it's standard operating procedure. And it disconnects us from life in the present.

There are many ways in which staying in the moment promotes health, healing, and recovery. My mind has to stop or at least slow way down before my heart can fully open. Staying in the moment provides me with freedom from the prisons of the past and fantasies of the future. It bestows respite from being trapped in the emotions associated with past events, such as resentment, guilt, shame, and regret, as well as those feelings linked with the future, primarily anxiety and fear. Everyone has a past, and it's okay and even healthy to visit it from time to time in order to better understand it, put it in perspective, and learn from it. And obviously, looking at and planning for the future is important and positive. It's when so much time is spent in the past or the future that our conscious focus is distracted from the here and now that it becomes problematic. Besides, until someone learns how to change the past, it's as good as it's ever going to get. It's impossible to change what happened yesterday or know with any certainty what will happen tomorrow.

When we aren't paying conscious attention to the present moment, we are effectively sleepwalking, even when we are wide awake. When we're focused on the past or the future, we are cut off from the possibilities inherent in this moment—unable to see it and experience it for what it is; separated from the opportunities it presents. We may be with someone physically, but somewhere else and perhaps with someone else mentally and emotionally.

As present-centering as sports can be for me, when I'm not in the moment, my performance is affected. When I'm playing tennis, but mired in upset about hitting the last point out of bounds, it's much harder for me to play the current point skillfully. If I'm in the middle of a bowling game and I'm worried about what my final score will be, my focus is distracted from the ball I'm rolling right now.

How many times have you been driving and missed your intended turn or exit, or came close to missing it, because you weren't paying enough attention to the here and now? How many fender benders and other more serious traffic accidents occur because drivers are mentally somewhere else, not focused on the present moment? This is instructive of how not being present-centered can interfere with attention and performance to the point where it becomes a form of impairment.

Fortunately, the potential for learning, growing, and healing exists in each and every moment. Even though we may have spent the last few minutes somewhere else—in the past or the future—as soon as we become aware of it, we can make a conscious choice to shift our focus to be present-centered in the here and now.

The value of conscious present-centered awareness, also known as mindfulness, is ancient wisdom, deriving from the spiritual traditions of Taoism in China in 600 BCE and Buddhism in India in 500 BCE. Shortly after I moved to LA in early 1977, a friend of my roommate gave me a copy of *Remember, Be Here Now* by Ram Dass, saying, "You're ready for this." Before the author became Ram Dass, yogi and spiritual teacher, he was Richard Alpert, PhD, a prominent psychologist at Harvard University. At Harvard, Alpert's explorations of human consciousness led him to conduct intensive research with LSD and other psychedelic substances in collaboration with fellow Harvard psychologist Timothy Leary. Because of the highly controversial nature of their research, both were fired from Harvard in 1963.

Leary and Alpert had determined that the use of psychedelic drugs was a direct route to spiritual enlightenment, and their goal was to find a way to remain in an ongoing LSD-induced state of expanded consciousness. But no matter how much acid they took, it always wore off, ultimately leaving Alpert dissatisfied and despondent, and sparking an alternative quest for spirituality that led him to question many of his assumptions about himself and life. In 1967, he traveled to India where he met his spiritual teacher or guru. So spiritually evolved was this individual that even a monstrous dose of the purest LSD seemed to have no effect on him, because he was "already there."

Alpert embarked on a rigorous path of spiritual study and practice that included meditation, yoga, and *pranayama* (focused intentional breathing practices) that led to his transformation to Baba Ram Dass. His mission became to make Eastern spirituality more accessible to Western culture. *Remember, Be Here Now*, first published in 1971, was a groundbreaking manifestation of that mission. At the heart of this trance-inducing work is the transformative power of a conscious appreciation of the present moment and the importance of remaining centered in it.

Among its array of consciousness-raising content, *Remember, Be Here Now* explained the value of intentional silence and the direct connection between silence and present-centered awareness/mindfulness. I was intrigued to the point that one evening a week after work I practiced maintaining personal silence, not speaking at all as a means to enhance my conscious contact with the moment. As strange as it felt initially, it quickly became comfortable. And it was wonderfully effective, imparting a spiritual centeredness I had never experienced before. However, for my roommate and our friends who came over to party regardless of the day or the time, it was weird as shit. I continued this practice for about five months before letting it go. I have yet to return to it.

Mindfulness is a state of awareness based on paying conscious attention to one's internal and external experience. It creates a receptive space in which one observes thoughts, feelings, and bodily sensations as they are, without judging or trying to suppress or deny them. It is direct contact, unobstructed by thoughts and judgments, with ourselves and the world around us. Mindfulness practice cultivates the ability to observe and accept the ongoing unfolding of one's experience without becoming over-identified with or attached to the content of thoughts, emotions, and sensory experiences. It stimulates the recognition that thoughts and feelings come and go of their own accord.

This is especially relevant for people struggling with addiction and/or chronic pain—mindfulness practice helps develop the skill of observing urges to avoid or suppress emotional and physical pain and ride these urges out, rather than act on them reflexively and unconsciously, often by using. Such urges to numb or escape by using are like waves on an ocean beach: they rise, crest, crash, and recede. By facilitating conscious awareness with a detached nonjudgmental perspective, mindfulness mitigates the tendency to get caught up in vicious circles of anxiety, fear, anger, guilt, regret, and shame that render those in recovery from addiction and/or chronic pain more vulnerable to using.

Mindfulness is the present-centered awareness that awakens the individual from the sleep of habitual responses—responses conditioned by beliefs and expectations with origins in the past that become projected onto the future. When I am in the default unconscious auto-pilot mode, the extent to which I can mentally manufacture stories about what might/could happen—having nothing whatsoever to do with the present moment—never ceases to amaze me, and these narratives are almost always worse (often much worse) then what actually happens. In the words of Mark Twain, "I have been through some terrible things in my life, some of which actually happened."

Through mindfulness and its associated practice of meditation, people develop a greater capacity to face uncomfortable, painful thoughts, feelings, and physical sensations, learning simply to accept the pain, anxiety, anger, or sadness and let it pass, without obsessing on it or needing to change it. Research has demonstrated that the practice of mindfulness meditation leads to improvements in attention, concentration, openness to experience, ability to inhibit distracting stimuli, and perceptual sensitivity.[11] Mindfulness practice has also been shown to support the acceptance of thoughts and experiences as alternatives to attempting to avoid or suppress them.[12]

Active addiction, oriented as it is on immediate gratification by means of changing feelings, controlling people and situations, and tunnel-vision on where the next fix is coming from, is the antithesis of present-centered mindful acceptance. Consequently, nurturing conscious moment-to-moment awareness and developing the skills of mindfulness and meditation are among the cornerstones of a well-rounded skill-set that promotes long-term recovery. Although expanded awareness and acceptance of one's present experience is the proximate goal, increased calmness, contentment, and serenity often come about as by-products of practicing mindfulness and meditation.

Meditation is one of the main roads that leads to a state of mindfulness. I was fortunate to learn how to meditate when I was sixteen. At my mother's suggestion, my brother and I were trained in Transcendental Meditation (TM). She figured I could benefit from anything that might have a calming influence and wasn't a street drug, and it seemed interesting to me. Anything that could help bring some coherent semblance of centeredness and sanity to my trying-to-figure-out-who-the-hell-I-was-and-how-the-fuck-I-fit-in teenage self was worth checking out.

A month prior to the training we attended an introductory session on the philosophy and benefits of TM. The instructor stated that in order to get maximum benefit from the training, it was strongly recommended that participants not smoke pot for the two weeks prior to it. While my brother did this easily, I thought about it and said, "Fuck it," rationalizing that I could stop; I just didn't want to. I'll never know if or how continuing to smoke pot impacted my meditation, but I liked the experience of meditating immediately—it felt good, and I felt better after I did it. I meditated on a daily basis consistently for several years, and then on and off, before re-establishing a daily practice in my early to mid-thirties.

The mind is like a wild horse that utilizes its tremendous strength and energy indiscriminately. Much of its activity seems random, running in circles, bucking and kicking. Like a fart in the wind, it's all over the place. Meditation endeavors to train the mind so that gradually and progressively, its energy and strength can be harnessed and intentionally focused. Meditation accesses and conserves mental resources for conscious application.

The purpose of meditation is to bring us to this moment, here and now. There are many ways to meditate, and different types of meditation utilize distinctive vehicles to establish and maintain present-centered attention. Meditation approaches can be divided into two basic styles:

Concentrative practices are aimed at sustaining conscious attention on specific content, such as particular internal sounds or bodily sensations. Open awareness practices have a more broad-based focus, aiming to develop a big-picture monitoring ability in which sensory content and experience is registered, but not fixated upon.

Insight meditation (also known as mindfulness meditation) is an open awareness practice, while breathing meditation and mantra meditation are examples of concentrative practices. Insight meditation centers conscious attention on internal and external sensory stimuli using a relaxed though focused observation of thoughts, emotions, and bodily sensations as they arise and fall. Breathing meditation focuses on the breath—being consciously aware of your breathing, making that the locus of attention as you slowly and deeply breathe in on your inhale and out on your exhale. Mantra meditation concentrates conscious attention on a mantra, an energy-based sound that produces a specific physical vibration, and may or may not have any particular meaning. The word mantra means to free yourself from your mind. It originates from two Sanskrit words: *manas*, or mind, and *trai*, meaning to free from or liberate.

I practice Transcendental Meditation daily, using the mantra I was given during my original training. Intentionally focusing my awareness on this sound and repeating it internally in sync with the rhythm of my breathing enables me to sustain conscious contact with the present moment. However, from time to time, I also practice mindfulness meditation to further enhance my conscious present-centeredness.

Meditation quiets the mind, helping still the thoughts that continuously wash over it. A common question of people beginning meditation is "how do I stop my thoughts?" The answer is, you don't. The desire to "stop" thoughts mobilizes both resistance and judgment, and works against meditation's fundamental intent. Even during meditation, other thoughts—including those related to the past or future—intrude on this most conscious and disciplined effort to stay in the moment.

I have a choice to make in how I respond to such "intrusions." While I could become frustrated, angry, or self-critical (and early in my meditation practice I did), I strive to accept them without judging either the thoughts or myself. It is a natural phenomenon for thoughts of other things to creep in to the best efforts to remain present-centered. This is neither positive nor negative; it simply is. When thoughts encroach, I've learned to observe them without becoming attached to them. I can note their presence, like birds flying by overhead, without letting them make nests in my hair or crap on my head. I become consciously aware that my mind has drifted away from the moment, and use that awareness to matter-of-factly refocus my attention on my mantra, which brings me back to the here and now.

Oftentimes my meditation process works beautifully—exquisitely deep and calming, suffusing me with serenity and spirituality, intimately connecting me with both my internal experience and that which is beyond myself. On other occasions, not so much. There are days when it feels superficial and ineffective as my attention seems to wander from one thought to another throughout the session. Even with many years of experience there is considerable variation in the "purity" and quality of my meditation practice. Experience has taught me to accept this as part of the process and to continue my practice daily—whether the external environment is conducive to meditation or not, and whether my internal environment is relaxed and calm or anxious and stressed.

Although there can be significant immediate benefits to meditation and mindfulness practice, the positive effects are also cumulative over time. Recent research using functional magnetic resonance imaging (fMRI) finds that meditation produces positive changes in the brain's ability to process emotions that endure even when people are not actively meditating.[13] Small pebbles can create big ripples. This is a gift that I give to myself.

Stress affects everyone. It plays a major role in many physical and emotional illnesses; numerous medical conditions are caused or exacerbated by stress. According to the Centers for Disease Control and Prevention, up to 90 percent of doctor visits in the US may be related to stress. Meditation and mindfulness practice are effective antidotes for stress, calming the nervous system by activating the relaxation response, a set of physiological processes that offset the physiological effects of stress.

In stimulating the relaxation response (the physiological opposite of the "fight or flight" response), meditation flips a switch that turns on the parasympathetic division of the autonomic nervous system (ANS). The parasympathetic division is involved in rest, relaxation, recharge, and conservation of energy. Upon its activation, breathing slows and deepens, muscles soften, metabolism and pulse rate slow, and blood pressure decreases.

The health benefits of meditation and mindfulness practice are wide-ranging and have been documented by scientific research for over thirty years. In addition to decreasing stress with all of the secondary health gains that come with that, meditation has a protective impact on heart health by contributing to measurable decreases in cardiac risk factors. Empirical studies have demonstrated that meditation practice can help: reduce high cholesterol;[14] reduce insulin resistance, glucose, and even insulin levels themselves;[15] reduce blood pressure and hypertension;[16] and reduce the risk of heart disease and stroke among individuals over the age of fifty-five.[17]

Similar to keeping a fine instrument properly tuned, meditation practice enriches the brain's neuronal structures, enhances connections, and affects neurotransmitter levels positively by decreasing those related to stress and arousal—cortisol and norepinephrine, and increasing those involved in relaxation and mood regulation—serotonin and GABA.[18] When we exercise parts of the brain, which occurs during meditation, they become larger and denser with neural mass or gray matter.

Studies also indicate meditation has neuroprotective effects, mitigating some of the impacts of aging. The volume of the brain's gray matter ordinarily diminishes with age. However, scientists found that in meditators (in contrast to a comparison group of non-meditators), the volume of gray matter hadn't reduced at all with age.[19] Follow-up research suggests that long-term meditators also have stronger connections between different parts of the brain while finding less age-related decline in the brain's white-matter tissue.[20]

Moreover, meditation can help people face physical pain more successfully. A study using magnetic resonance imaging technology that captures longer duration brain processes (ASL MRI) showed that meditation can dramatically reduce both the experience of pain and pain-related brain activation.[21] Meditation expands the ability to consciously shift the perception of pain, and better accept the pain that is experienced, without obsessing over or trying to change it.

Mindfulness-based applications that incorporate meditation have been developed for a wide range of behavioral health problems and populations. Empirically supported treatments that are based on or incorporate mindfulness training include: Acceptance and Commitment Therapy; Dialectical Behavior Therapy; Mindfulness-Based Cognitive Therapy; and Mindfulness-Based Stress Reduction. Mindfulness-based protocols have also been developed for relapse prevention for addictive behaviors. With over 2,500 years of history and an expanding and compelling body of scientific research behind it, more medical and behavioral health professionals are incorporating mindfulness practices into their approaches to helping people.

Meditation and mindfulness practice become even more important in a world that is increasingly Attention Deficit Disorder-inducing, with seductive distractions constantly demanding our attention, normalizing unrealistic breadths of multitasking, and spreading ourselves more and more thin. Our technology-driven culture, with its twenty-four/seven connectivity via the proliferation of new mobile information technology and social networking platforms, places ever-greater demands on our time, energy, attention, and emotional availability.

How common has it become for people to be plugged in to their smart phones, tablets, and other devices, absorbed in electronic pacification, completely disassociated from where they are and who they are with? Sometimes even during meditation, when my smart phone signals that a new text or email has arrived and awaits my attention, I'm automatically drawn to it. Conscious awareness that the incessant accessibility of digital information and virtual communication represents an ongoing threat to present-centered being is essential to steering me away from the pull of its allure. But I need to follow up this awareness with action. I have to exercise the skills I've developed to stay in the moment and not pick up the goddamn phone. Of course, turning it off for the duration of this or any other activity is also an option.

In my twelve-step program we often talk about the importance of staying in the moment. Replaying the past or fantasizing about the future impairs anyone's ability to be skillful in the present, but for those of us in recovery, getting stuck in those places mentally and emotionally has special risks. There are a number of ways in which twelve-step recovery literature addresses the value of meditation, but the Eleventh Step places particular emphasis on it.

I have an abiding appreciation for each of the Twelve Steps, but the Eleventh Step has special resonance for me. There are two parts to Step Eleven. The first is about using meditation (and prayer) to improve our conscious contact with that which is greater than ourselves—our individually defined higher power. Conscious contact with this higher power (whatever that may be for us) creates connection with the commonalities we share; the ties that link humankind, the world, and the universe together, and diffuses that which separates us from ourselves, from each other, and from nature.

As the stresses of modern life compel people to engage with the world at higher speeds while being pulled in more different directions, most drift further away from any mindful consideration of the present moment, and from the values that are truly important to them. The second part of the

Eleventh Step speaks to letting life happen of its own accord and going with its natural current, instead of swimming against its flow and trying to force it to comply with my desires. Practicing Step Eleven is instrumental in uncovering and recovering those priorities that are most important to me and that are integral to assembling a life of value and meaning.

Through the daily practice of mindfulness and meditation I settle more fully and comfortably into my own skin, and experience conscious connectedness with others, along with the sources of my spiritual sustenance. Being present-centered in the moment gives me sanctuary from the cocoon of self-absorption where ruminations about past wrongs perpetrated by or upon me, and future worries about what might happen to me or those I care about run rampant.

There are certain places—in the literal, geographic sense—that are portals to present-centeredness. They routinely transport me to a keen awareness of the here and now, capturing my conscious attention, anchoring me in the moment. It is easy for my heart to be at peace in the mountains or at the beach where the immensity of the big trees and massive rock formations or the enormity of the ocean hypnotizes and humbles, and the sweet softness of the wind whistling through the forest and lilting lullaby of the waves bathe my soul in serenity.

In such awe-inspiring environments, conscious contact with that which is beyond oneself; with God as I understand that concept, abounds. The imaginary line between me and the rest of nature melts away, connecting me directly and intimately to the wider world around me and my place within it. Wilderness hiking is a walking meditation, firmly holding my attention, as my perspective oscillates between the big-picture panorama and the immediacy of the trail's next step, allowing me to see both the forest and its trees.

The hamster wheel in my head slows and fades, leaving only presence. For long moments, as all else disappears, I may be aware of nothing more than the muted kaleidoscope of colors embedded in boulders of granite, the well-defined striations in walls of red rock sandstone, the rough-hewn charcoal-gray bark of a Douglas Fir, the flaky light-brown-amber trunk of a Ponderosa Pine, or the gnarled corkscrew branches of Bristlecone Pines that only grow above 9,000 feet in the mountains of southern Nevada and live to up to 4,000 years. In the wilderness, my mind, heart, and spirit become one, and merge with everything around me.

John Muir, the visionary naturalist, who discovered the wonders of the Sierra Nevada and Yosemite Valley and its surrounding wilderness in the late nineteenth century and cofounded the Sierra Club wrote, "Climb the mountains and get their good tidings. Nature's peace will flow into you as sunshine flows into trees. The winds will blow their own freshness into you, and the storms their energy, while cares will drop off like autumn leaves."[22] "Beauty beyond thought everywhere, beneath, above, made and being made forever."[23]

It is only through being present-centered that I am genuinely mentally, emotionally, and spiritually available. When I'm able and content to simply be here now, my heart is accessible to the values that hold meaning for me. When I live fully in this moment, I have the capacity to get out of my own way and open myself to whatever learning, growing, and healing the moment has to offer. And yet, as long as I've been practicing, I still often stray, however briefly, into the past or the future. Staying in the moment with awareness and acceptance is an ongoing challenge. As part of my mindfulness practice, I use several different mantras (outside of my meditation), along with deep breathing through my nose and into my abdomen to refocus my attention consciously, and I regularly remind myself to "be here now." Much like recovery itself, staying in the moment is a process, rather than an event.

chapter fifteen

[PAIN IS INEVITABLE;]
SUFFERING IS OPTIONAL

*"Between stimulus and response there is a space. In
that space is our power to choose our response. In our
response lies our growth and our freedom."*
VIKTOR FRANKL

In *Man's Search for Meaning*, Viktor Frankl, a Jewish psychiatrist, wrote about the psychological impacts of life as a prisoner in the Nazi concentration camps of World War II. His mother, father, brother, and pregnant wife were all killed in the camps. Dr. Frankl describes in chilling detail how his captors took from him virtually everything of personal value and basic human dignity. The only thing that the Nazis were unable to take away was his choice as to how to respond to the deprivation, degradation, and trauma to which he was subjected. He made a conscious decision to focus his energies on "owning" that small but all-important space between the stimulus (whatever was said or done to him) and his response to it. His ability to retain that degree of psycho-spiritual autonomy in the most horrific circumstances imaginable provides a remarkable example of intrapersonal strength, grace under extreme duress, the power of personal choice, and the Serenity Prayer in action.

Although Buddhism predates the establishment of Western psychology and psychotherapy, and twelve-step recovery by well over two millennia, these three distinct provinces—spiritual, professional, and self-help— share certain underlying commonalities in theory and practice. Most importantly for our purposes, each of them represent approaches to understanding and ameliorating suffering, and all three offer pathways toward transformation and healing.

In the *Diagnostic and Statistical Manual of Mental Disorders* (DSM), there are hundreds of diagnosable conditions. Each of them is conceptualized as a clinically significant behavioral or psychological syndrome or pattern that causes current distress (such as painful symptoms) or disability (impairment in one or more important areas of functioning)—in other words, suffering. Behavioral health treatment, including psychotherapy, exists to help people find relief from their suffering and lead healthier, more satisfying lives.

The Four Noble Truths of Buddhism address suffering as innate to the human condition. The First Truth is that suffering is a part of life. Suffering in all its forms represents lack of satisfaction/contentment/ fulfillment. The Second Truth is that suffering is caused and exacerbated by attachment to/desire for something different than "what is." This includes having things we don't want, as well as wanting things we don't have. The Third Truth is that, though a part of life, suffering is not inevitable. And the Fourth Truth is that there are paths out of suffering.

The Buddhist way out of suffering is the mindfulness-focused Eightfold Path: 1) Right Understanding, Right View; 2) Right Aspiration, Right Thinking; 3) Right Speech; 4) Right Action; 5) Right Livelihood; 6) Right Effort; 7) Right Mindfulness; 8) Right Concentration. Twelve-step programs provide another such pathway that in many respects parallels the principles of the Eightfold Path.

From an early age, through effectively downloading data from everything we observe and experience, we are conditioned to categorize experiences, including emotions and physical sensations, in terms of whether they are "good" or "bad." Sadness, anxiety, fear, and physical pain are viewed as bad or negative, while happiness, joy, and being pain-free are perceived as good or positive. Consequently, it becomes natural to want to avoid experiences judged to be bad, negative, or painful. When we experience pain, whether the source of that pain is emotional or physical, we generally attempt to avoid it. After all, who wants to be in pain?

As discussed earlier, addiction frequently originates as a way to escape from, numb, and ultimately avoid pain via mood-altering substances or behaviors (such as gambling, eating, and sex) that then become reinforced and habituated through repetition. Ironically, these efforts to keep emotional and physical pain at bay end up creating even more of it. Avoidance doesn't work because pain is an inevitable part of life. It is an essential aspect of being human. Everyone experiences uncomfortable, painful thoughts, emotions, and physical sensations. Avoiding pain is quite simply impossible. It is in how we choose to respond to the emotional and physical pain we experience that determines whether we are able to get through that pain, or unwittingly extend and amplify it.

For those who struggle with addiction and/or chronic pain, at times the challenges of living can seem insurmountable. Chronic pain has many of the same adverse bio-psycho-social-spiritual impacts as active addiction, including: damage to relationships—such as primary relationships, marriages, parent-child, family, and friendships, and job/career and financial problems, along with impairments in eating, sleeping, and mood. Discouragement, fear, isolation, feelings of inadequacy and worthlessness, depression, grief/loss, desperation, guilt, shame, and often self-loathing ensue from the experience of being enslaved by debilitating repetitive behaviors and chronic conditions. These emotions generate yet another layer of pain to fend off, ratcheting up reliance on avoidance strategies that are doomed to fail.

Trying to escape painful thoughts, feelings, and physical sensations may work temporarily, but in the long run it only prolongs those experiences and intensifies the suffering connected to them. Suffering is a function of how people think and feel about the emotional and physical pain they experience, and the beliefs they attach to it. Whenever the belief exists that someone shouldn't be in pain or that pain is something to be avoided at all costs, and in turn they feel angry or depressed about being in pain, then that person will experience suffering. There is a direct correlation between the amount of effort expended to avoid pain and the degree of suffering experienced—the harder someone works to avoid pain, the greater his or her suffering tends to be.

Physical pain conditions should *always* be assessed by medical professionals. That being said, there are substantial differences between pain management—the conventional medicalized approach to treating pain, and a bio-psycho-social-spiritual approach known as Pain Recovery. Pain management is a paradigm driven by doctors and the healthcare system, the primary goal of which is to control, if not eliminate, pain. This is a more recent subspecialty of medicine. Most pain management specialists are trained as anesthesiologists, whose primary training is to put patients to sleep, literally. These physicians usually go through a fellowship training program to learn prevailing Western medical techniques to treat pain.

Pain management involves prescribing opioid pain medications that often distort thinking and judgment, and, as I've exemplified, can be highly addictive. Pain management relies on physical interventions that range from less invasive to more invasive, such as physical therapy, steroid injections, nerve blocks, and surgeries in order to eliminate or decrease pain. Obviously, invasive procedures have their own risks, some of which are considerable. Pain management sometimes uses treatment modalities that are less traditional and minimally invasive, such as: acupuncture, chiropractic, massage, and hydrotherapy, among others. These less invasive treatments, known as Complementary and Alternative Medicine (CAM), are also commonly utilized as part of an alternative approach to chronic pain: pain recovery.

By reinforcing the illusion that pain can be eliminated or controlled, the pain management process inadvertently increases suffering. With most chronic pain conditions, though the pain may wax and wane, it rarely goes away. Therefore, the goal of eliminating pain altogether is, in the great majority of cases, simply not realistic.

The basis of pain recovery is giving up the quest to have pain to disappear. Its goals are to learn ways to accept the existence of pain, develop the skills to live with it rather than attempting to numb or escape it, and improve functioning. This approach is designed to equip those afflicted with chronic pain to address their pain in healthier ways, and gain freedom from thinking, feeling, and acting like a victim, without the use of opioids or other habit-forming substances.

Pain recovery is a solution-focused approach to treating chronic pain that encompasses mental, emotional, and spiritual, in addition to physical functioning. Chronic pain is like an smoke detector that goes on and becomes stuck in the "on" mode, continuously sounding a harrowing alarm at high volume. Pain recovery distinguishes between the actual pain and the suffering it causes, and focuses on achieving relief from suffering. Pain is unavoidable; suffering is not. It occurs in response to thoughts such as "Why me?" "It isn't fair!" "This is horrible!" "I can't stand it!" along with the spectrum of distressing emotions associated with pain.

As mentioned in Chapter Eight, Dr. Mel Pohl is a nationally recognized expert on chronic pain and addiction as co-occurring disorders. Dr. Pohl is the principal developer of the pain recovery model. He views suffering—

the cognitive and emotional responses to pain that perpetuate and exacerbate it—as the true target of intervention. According to Dr. Pohl, an analysis of how patients in the LVRC Pain Recovery Program described their pain suggests that approximately 80 percent of it relates to suffering.

Suffering in general, as well as specific to addiction and/or chronic pain, is a function of imbalances in physical, mental, emotional, physical, and/or spiritual functioning. Recovery is a gradual, progressive, and ongoing process of restoring balance in these areas. Suffering is both a cause and an effect of the full range of emotions associated with chronic pain—anxiety, irritability, anger, fear, depression, frustration, guilt, shame, loneliness, hopelessness, and perceived helplessness. Pain recovery involves the way we think, how we respond to feelings, our physical functioning, and our spirituality, and applies the time-tested efficacy of the principles of the Twelve Steps to the challenges of living with chronic pain.

Scientific study continually generates proof of the intimate connections between the mind and body, with empirical research on meditation and mindfulness practices cited in the previous chapter providing compelling evidence of this linkage. Whatever affects the mind or the body will inevitably affect the other, regardless of which side of the fence an issue originates. As a result, imbalances in thinking can contribute to imbalances in physical, emotional, and spiritual functioning.

Negative thinking only makes situations we believe to be "bad," worse. Many people, including those who do not suffer from addiction or chronic pain, can ruminate on something by continuously and unproductively replaying it in their minds or magnify the negative aspects of it, exaggerating its significance, and turning what was really only a small problem into a major disaster in their minds.

Whenever I emphasize the negative aspects of my experience by the way I think about them, my mood goes south and I make my life more negative. Our thoughts have the capacity to make us miserable, and negative thinking can be especially insidious, feeding on itself, with the potential to become a self-fulfilling, self-defeating prophesy. It is important to be aware that if negative thought patterns are not addressed, they lead to negative, unhealthy behaviors—for addicts that often means an eventual return to active addiction.

For people with chronic pain, there is a direct correlation between negative thinking and beliefs, and the level of pain they experience—the more negative the thoughts and beliefs, the greater the pain sensations and the more intense the urges to numb, escape, or avoid them. This quickly becomes a vicious circle as pain triggers negative thoughts and internal self-talk (what we tell ourselves about our pain), then translates to feelings that coincide with suffering, and increases muscle tension and stress, which in turn, amplify the pain signals, triggering more of them.

The progression is essentially as follows: pain leads to negative thoughts/self-talk/beliefs lead to feelings of frustration/anger/anxiety/ fear/sadness/depression/hopelessness lead to suffering leads to muscle tension and stress lead to more pain leads to increased negative thoughts/self-talk/beliefs lead to increased frustration/anger/anxiety/ fear/sadness/depression/hopelessness leads to greater suffering, and so on. The longer such a cycle continues, the more out of balance a person becomes.

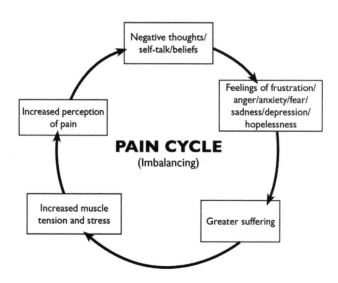

Suffering can be modified when people learn how to respond differently to their pain. The process of pain recovery includes dramatically changing this negative progression starting with regaining balance in thinking through the application of mindfulness-based practices. Reestablishing balance counteracts the above deviation-amplifying dynamics: conscious awareness of negative thinking/self-talk and how it sets off the cascade of events that fuels suffering leads to mindful acceptance and detached observation of negative thinking/self-talk lead to minimization/elimination of suffering leads to decreased feelings of frustration/anger/anxiety/fear/sadness/depression/hopelessness leads to lower stress and muscle tension leads to less pain.

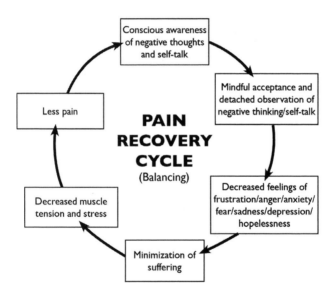

By adjusting my thinking, and how I think about my thinking, it is possible to change my emotional responses, the extent to which I suffer (or not), my level of tension and stress, and in turn, my experience of pain. The premise that thoughts have significant effects on feelings and behavior and that shifts in thinking lead to emotional and behavioral changes is the basis of Cognitive Behavioral Therapy (CBT). This knowledge has an extensive history, having been a topic of discussion among Stoic philosophers in ancient Greece and Rome (notably Epictetus and Marcus Aurelius).

CBT techniques are used to help individuals identify their maladaptive cognitive patterns and beliefs, such as discounting the positive in a situation by focusing on the negative; blowing things out of proportion; thinking in rigid black-and-white/all-or-nothing extremes; and placing unreasonable and unrealistic expectations on oneself, other people, and situations—"I *should* be better than this," "This traffic *must* go faster." (I've learned how not to "should" all over myself, and I'm no longer a habitual "must"erbator.) Getting caught in these cognitive traps escalates emotional pain and invariably gooses the experience of suffering.

CBT seeks to replace such distorted thinking with more realistic and effective thoughts to reduce emotional distress and self-defeating behaviors. The process of replacing problematic cognitions with those that are more healthy and adaptive is referred to as cognitive restructuring. Cognitive restructuring is sometimes contrasted with cognitive defusion—a related but divergent set of techniques that draw on mindfulness practices and are emphasized in Acceptance and Commitment Therapy (ACT). ACT is an evidence-based adaptation of CBT that features mindfulness and internal values-congruent practices. While the aim of cognitive restructuring is to actively change distressing thoughts and patterns of thinking, cognitive defusion focuses on observing and accepting uncomfortable thoughts without automatically buying into or attaching any particular value to them. Cognitive restructuring and cognitive defusion share a common foundation of bringing unhealthy automatic thinking to conscious awareness. They each change the nature of the relationship we have with our thoughts and thought process. Both of them have been important parts of my pain recovery process, though increasingly I gravitate toward mindfulness-based techniques.

Through awareness and practice anyone struggling with chronic pain can develop the skills to disengage from the habitual unconscious cognitive routines that activate suffering. Learning to recognize pain-related patterns of negative thinking and relate to them more adaptively through constructive disengagement—viewing them as passing events in the mind—diffuses the influence of those patterns. Deepening awareness and nonjudgmental acceptance of one's thoughts fosters a new relationship with them, creating the space to purposefully shift mental focus away from the ruminative thought patterns that pave the road to suffering. For those struggling with addiction, the upcoming exit on that road may well be relapse.

Thoughts occur so naturally and automatically that we are oriented to see them as part of ourselves. We become so closely identified with our thoughts that we believe there is no separation; our thoughts are us and we are our thoughts. And yet, the reality is that we produce our thoughts; they are mental products generated in our minds.

We are also inclined to believe in the inherent truth or accuracy of our thoughts. Assuming our thoughts are facts—that they are all true and valid without examination—is one of the reasons we often find ourselves out of balance. This is particularly true when people are challenged with chronic pain and/or addiction. Self-talk is an off-shoot of our thinking and refers to what we tell ourselves about events—both internal and external. Our self-talk defines our beliefs about those events. The more consciously aware of this process we become, the more we are able to develop the capacity to accept and, if we chose to, intentionally adjust our thinking, self-talk, and beliefs.

Thoughts are like images on the video screen of the mind. The first thoughts that come into your mind are like the channel that the television is turned to when you first turn the power on. While I may be powerless over the automatic thoughts that first enter my mind, I am not powerless over what I do in response to them. When I turn on the TV, I observe the channel that's on and notice its content. Then I make a decision to take some sort of action in response to it. It's important to be aware that no action is an action unto itself, and not making a decision is, in fact, making a decision by default. I can choose to leave the channel where it is, or if I don't care for what's on, I can lower the volume, mute the sound altogether, or change the channel to something more to my preference. In the same way, as I become more consciously aware of my thoughts, I can witness them without judgment; accept them with detachment and let them pass; question their accuracy; and/or dispute or challenge them, or modify them. Awareness opens up the possibility of multiple options that give me the power of conscious choice.

In pain recovery, with the aid of mindfulness practice, we learn that we are not what we think. We have thoughts; however, we are not our thoughts. We can observe them without identifying with them, and we can dispute them by not buying everything they are trying to sell us. Progress toward healing and recovery from chronic pain also requires acceptance that, although we cannot control our thoughts, we nonetheless have choices about how to respond to them and how much influence to accord them. Paying attention to our thought process and consciously observing, questioning, and challenging our thinking are indications of mental health. Mental balance involves moving away from rigid unconscious patterns of thinking and developing flexibility (open-mindedness) in how I think and how I think about my thought processes.

In an earlier chapter I described how my emotional and my physical pain fed each other to the point where they merged together to form this amorphous beast that precipitated immense suffering. I felt angry because it hurt so fucking much; I felt depressed because the pain seemed to never take time off; I felt sad because I couldn't be as physically active as I wanted; I felt fearful about what my pain condition meant for my future functioning; and I felt hopeless because there seemed to be little I could do to get better. And all of these emotional responses to my pain made it that much harder to bear. Pain recovery helps me distinguish between the emotional and physical components of my pain, use existing and newly acquired skills in response to my emotional pain, and reduce my suffering.

In recovery from addiction and chronic pain, emotional healing starts when I begin to connect consciously with and accept my feelings. Trying to avoid or suppress painful emotions is similar to being mired in quicksand. The harder I struggle to get free, the more stress and tension I create, the deeper I sink and the more stuck I become. It is only when I stop judging and struggling and allow what is there to simply be, that I can free myself, as distressing feelings lose their grip and dissipate on their own.

Feelings always find a path to expression. If I don't allow myself to feel them and, as necessary, talk about them; if I avoid or suppress those feelings, then they invariably come out "sideways"—in indirect forms via my behavior. When feelings are expressed through behavior, they typically operate unconsciously, outside of my awareness and ability to steward. When this happens I'm on autopilot, doing things I don't want to do and that I know won't work for me, but have no idea why I keep doing them.

It's similar to a pressure cooker. Pressure cookers are instruments of balance inasmuch as a lid is required to keep the contents from spilling all over the place, but a means to release the accumulating pressure is also necessary. If there is no release valve to provide it a safe path to expression, what happens? The pressure builds up until the vessel can no longer contain it and it explodes, causing potentially serious damage. In the same way, if I do not provide my feelings a safe (though at times uncomfortable) path to expression by feeling and talking about them consciously, they will still find a way out often through some sort of unhealthy, self-defeating and/or explosive behavior.

Feelings, especially powerful disturbing ones, can seem as though they will last forever. However, whether they are positive and bring smiles to our face and laughter to our lips, or painful and bring hurt to our hearts and tears to our eyes, feelings are *always* temporary. They come and go like guests who come to visit: some are welcome and we're delighted to see them; others, not so much. Sometimes they leave sooner than we would like; other times they stay way past the point when we want them to leave—but eventually they all leave. As we say in twelve-step recovery, "this too shall pass."

Dialectical Behavior Therapy (DBT) is an evidence-based cognitive behaviorally oriented treatment approach that blends a problem-solving focus with emotional regulation, distress tolerance, acceptance, and mindfulness strategies. DBT was originally developed to treat people with borderline personality disorder and those who are acutely suicidal—populations that are extremely emotionally intense and labile. These individuals are unable to manage feelings internally and are frequently intensely angry, frustrated, depressed, or anxious.

Many people struggling with chronic pain and/or addiction present with an emotional hypersensitivity—a pronounced difficulty tolerating painful feelings. This heightened sensitivity means emotions are felt more deeply and rapidly than by most other people. As a result, distressing feelings such as anxiety, fear, anger, guilt, shame, sadness, and depression, as well as physical pain are not only felt with great intensity, they are often experienced as overwhelming, almost suffocating. Using substances becomes a way to turn down the volume of such feelings and to numb them in order to survive them.

Distress tolerance is about enduring and accepting discomfort, learning to bear pain skillfully. Distress tolerance skills are an outgrowth of mindfulness practices, and involve the ability to nonjudgmentally accept both oneself and the current situation in spite of the emotional and physical distress experienced. It is important to clarify that acceptance does not equate to approval. We can learn to tolerate thoughts, emotions, physical sensations, and situations that we don't like at all, and may even deeply dislike. Distress tolerance enhances coping capacity by strengthening resiliency—the ability to adjust to change.

Emotional regulation relates to identifying the emotions that are being felt in the moment, and observing them without being overwhelmed by them. Emotional regulation skills include self-soothing techniques that provide a calming effect. These are self-care activities that help to reduce emotional intensity such as meditation, deep breathing, listening to music you enjoy, progressive muscle relaxation, taking a walk, reading something pleasurable or spiritual, singing a favorite song, exercising, visualizing a comforting/relaxing image, journaling, etc. Emotional regulation is aimed at modulating feelings in order to strengthen the capacity to manage impulses so as to not behave in reactive, self-defeating, and destructive ways.

Allowing oneself to feel, accept, express, and coexist with uncomfortable, often painful emotions is essential to recovery from chronic pain and addiction. Feeling and accepting emotions also takes less energy than running from or stifling them, making more energy available for recovery-supportive pursuits. Emotional balance is achievable when we allow ourselves to feel whatever comes up, without suppressing or being overwhelmed by it, and learn to accept those feelings without judgment.

Because my feelings are a part of me, accepting them as they are is integral to the process of accepting myself as I am. Many people struggle with self-acceptance, but those afflicted with chronic pain and/or addiction incur extraordinary challenges. This lack of self-acceptance is another factor that contributes to suffering. Hence, recovery involves progress toward being fundamentally okay with oneself. Whatever positive changes you want to make in your life, acceptance of how and where you are in the present moment is one of the keys to moving forward.

Dialectical thinking is based on the view that all things are interconnected and even elements that seem to be the antitheses of one another share a relationship. Dialectic is a dynamic process wherein apparent opposites move toward an integration that brings them into harmony and creates a greater whole. Pain recovery, the Twelve Steps, DBT, and ACT all utilize the dialectic of acceptance and change, recognizing the therapeutic value of accepting one's current status *and* moving toward healthy change to generate growth and healing. This dialectic is elegantly encapsulated in the Serenity Prayer:

Grant me the serenity to **accept** *the things I cannot change;*

The courage to **change** *the things I can;*

And the **wisdom** *to know the difference.*

One of the resources I draw on regularly in my recovery is the application of the Serenity Prayer and its dialectical dynamics. Everything I encounter in life ultimately breaks down into two categories: things that I can change or at least have some influence over, and things I cannot change or influence. If I take the time and make the space to consider it consciously, all of my experiences, both internal and external, fit into one of these two basic categories.

Simply recognizing which grouping a challenge at hand (be it physical, mental, emotional, spiritual, or interactional) belongs in makes my life more manageable. Beyond that, if the challenge is something I cannot change—such as the fact of being in pain or the actions or attitude of another person—I need to accept it, and the issue becomes how best to facilitate that acceptance. If, on the other hand, the challenge is something I can change—how I'm responding to the pain I have or how I'm dealing with that other person—the issue is about what I need to change and how to most effectively make it happen. One thing that I can always change (as difficult as it can be at times) is how I respond to that which I cannot change.

Although my introduction to twelve-step recovery was specific to my addiction, I've found that its principles and practices successfully generalize to a range of life challenges, including chronic pain. Working the twelve-step program as the foundation of my addiction recovery process has only strengthened my capacity to live with my chronic pain condition. It has given me access to multiple strategies and tools that I use to better tolerate emotional and physical pain, and accept feelings of all kinds without acting on them in ways that make the situation worse and create suffering for myself or others.

My twelve-step program nurtures cognitive defusion to separate oneself from one's thought process, as well as cognitive restructuring to replace negative, unhealthy thoughts and beliefs with those that support recovery. It advances a framework for practicing new recovery-oriented behaviors and encourages connecting with others who share similar experiences for mutual identification, understanding, and support. Further, it encourages the development of positive spirituality and recommends the application of spiritual principles such as acceptance, tolerance, open-mindedness, perseverance, humility, and gratitude, as a means to diffuse self-centeredness, increase feelings of well-being, and prompt additional opportunities for conscious contact with that which is beyond oneself—of belonging to a greater whole, of connection to others, as well as to the world as a whole.

Prior to treatment, my thinking usually fed irrational beliefs about my pain: "I shouldn't have pain." "This is intolerable!" "I have to take more pain meds!" Through pain recovery, I've learned alternative ways to approach my pain, including how I think about it, interpret it, and react to it. As I learned in my clinical hypnotherapy training, all experiences have a specific structure. If that structure changes, so will the experience. The structure of my experience of pain includes how I think about it, the beliefs I attach to it, and how I react to it emotionally. By modifying that structure, my experience of pain has shifted dramatically.

I still have chronic pain. It is an onerous, dogged, often enervating presence in my life. In a word (or two), it blows. If I were to break it down percentage-wise, I'm in some degree of low-back pain 85–90 percent of the time—at least when I'm awake. Ten to fifteen percent of the time I am graced with the absence of pain, and that is always a great blessing. Approximately 65–70 percent of the time, my pain is the "normal" uncomfortable nagging dull ache; 10–15 percent of the time it's worse than usual, barking louder and cutting into my conscious awareness more noticeably; and 10 percent of the time it's really fucking bad, requiring me to be especially mindful in terms of how I take care of it. However, since I've been in recovery, my pain rarely debilitates me or dictates my activities (though it certainly influences them), and no longer controls my life.

The tone for my recovery from addiction and chronic pain is set each day during the extensive multimodal early morning practice I described in the previous chapter, combining spiritual reading, meditation, nondenominational prayer, self-hypnosis, Egoscue stretching, and chi kung exercises. I do continue to utilize certain aspects of conventional Western and complementary alternative medicine, including ibuprophen, to mitigate pain and inflammation, and the targeted use of ice packs and heating pads, which besides helping to decrease pain sensations and deflect my attention from them, have the therapeutic benefits of reducing swelling and increasing blood circulation respectively. I have intermittent chiropractic and massage treatments, and have portable inferential stimulation and traction machines for home use as needed, though they rarely see the light of day.

One of the problems that comes with chronic pain is lack of movement. It can hurt too damn much to move, and the desire to protect oneself from pain is natural, so movement is often minimized and avoided as much as possible. Unfortunately, the less you move, the more pain you have when you do move, incentivizing you to move even less. It becomes one more vicious circle. Exercise consistent with one's capacity is an important part of the pain recovery process. Physical movement is the body's lubricant.

The more sedentary I am, the stiffer my back and other parts of my body become. There are times when I don't really want to move, and sure don't feel like moving, but knowing its therapeutic importance, I walk through my inertia. Currently, most of my workday is centered around my desk and usually on the computer. I make sure to get up and move around at least briefly every sixty to ninety minutes, and take a ten minute walk twice a day, even during the heat of the desert Southwest summer.

Pain recovery facilitates my ability to engage in positive behaviors and physical activities consistent with the internal values I hold dear, in spite of experiencing challenging thoughts, emotions, and physical sensations. In addition to experiencing noticeably less suffering, my physical functioning has increased markedly, though it's not without limitations. Subsequent to treatment, I started playing tennis for the first time in over thirty years. Tennis was actually a concession to my physical status and advancing "chronological maturity" in that I needed a primary aerobic athletic replacement for basketball (which is brutally hard on my back).

After entering recovery I also began to bowl in a league for the first since I was thirteen, and continue to do that weekly. I do mild to moderate strength training one to three times per week, and on rare occasions still shoot some hoops. I go hiking as often as I can, which, as I described, provides spiritual as well as physical exercise. I am aware that in return for participating in such activities and the joy they bring me, there will likely be some temporary increase in my pain level. I take the responsibility inherent in making a conscious decision to accept the cost-benefit trade-offs. I have learned to be attuned to shifting sands of my day-to-day, moment-to-moment physical capacity, and make adjustments in my overall schedule and participation in specific activities as necessary based on the signals my body sends.

Whenever I am present-centered in the moment and pay conscious attention to my internal and external experience—without trying to push away what feels bad or cling to what feels good—my relationship to pain changes. By turning toward the pain, accepting and embracing it rather than running away as fast as I can, my suffering diminishes and I am much more able to (more or less) gracefully accept my chronic pain and its impact on my life.

On Father's Day in 2010, after sleeping in to the luxuriously late hour of 7:00 a.m., I went on unconscious autopilot with regard to my lower back and it cost me big time. It began with the most ordinary and benign of exertions. I figured I'd empty the small waste baskets in the upstairs bedrooms and bathrooms on my way downstairs en route to my usual first activities upon waking: making coffee, checking email, and perusing the *New York Times* online.

Where I became mindless was in completely forgetting to pay attention to my body mechanics, specifically the positioning of my back. No doubt I took for granted that those waste baskets were oh-so-light (they contained only paper and weighed virtually nothing) it wouldn't matter that I was bending over in a way that put stress on a vulnerable part of my back. I knew better, but I forgot that I knew . . . until I felt the sickening twinge-pop and searing pain signals gushing from the area around my lumbar spine. I would have kicked myself in the ass if I was able to lift my leg, but since I was immobilized in blistering pain, beating the shit out of myself mentally and emotionally had to suffice.

By assuming that what I was doing was no big deal physically, and that I didn't need to consider it consciously, I had done some real damage. For several long moments, after more than three-and-a-half years in recovery, all I could think about was how much I wanted, needed, had to have some serious pain meds. Fuck the ibuprophen, gimme the opioids! My distorted and pain-addled thinking provided fertile soil for my suffering to take root.

I reached out for support and to vent through the twenty-first century vehicle of choice: social networking. So I posted my travails on Facebook, spawning posts of sympathy from friends across the country, and a rapid repartee with my friend Lew. Though we knew each other from Tucson, Lew had lived in close proximity to places where I had lived on both Long Island and in Rockland County, NY. At that time, he had nearly twenty years in recovery.

I concluded my initial post/rant with "I have a choice as to whether to continue to stew in this shit or try to see what it has to teach me and use it as an opportunity to practice some spirituality."

Lew: "Or maybe see a Dr.?"

Me: "Maybe, but not on a Father's Day Sunday my friend. Perhaps tomorrow, though I've been around this particular block often enough (too fucking often) to be able to do a pretty damn accurate assessment and I basically know the treatment protocols."

Lew: "Or maybe it has nothing to teach you? Maybe you just hurt your back? And maybe we don't need added opportunities to practice spirituality? Maybe we should just practice spirituality, period?"

Me: "If I was Buddha or Lao Tzu, I might know the answers to those questions, or maybe not."

Lew: "But if you were Buddha or Lao Tzu, you'd be dead this morning, so enjoy the day! Happy Father's Day."

Lew's humorous and sage sentiments gave me pause to step back from the situation's edge and brought a smile to my face at a time when I wouldn't have believed it possible. In the process, my suffering receded conspicuously.

The next day, my chiropractor, a specialist in sports medicine who once pitched in the College World Series gave me the diagnosis: severe sprain of the ligaments connecting the sacroiliac joint to the base of the spine. Prognosis: from the standpoint of recovery from the injury, fortunately excellent—as long as I took it easy and followed the recommended course of treatment and paid close and careful attention to my body mechanics and positioning. A caveat I knew well was that nasty sprains are notoriously vulnerable to re-injury and can also increase susceptibility to future injury. Treatment: lots of quality time in close contact with ice packs, increasing my ibuprophen intake, several chiropractic treatments, a little inferential electrical stimulation, and most importantly, avoidance of re-injury.

Outcome: I was in significant pain for a week, missed several days of work, and remained stiff and sore with attenuated mobility for nearly a month. However, I was back to about 80 percent of normal functioning within ten days. I missed two weeks of league bowling, but was back on the lanes eighteen days after the injury. I didn't bowl very well, but I was grateful to be able to bowl at all. My recuperation wasn't a straight line, but it continued without the need for any medication stronger than ibuprophen.

Contrary to one of Lew's comments, this episode did have some lessons for me. Clearly, operating unconsciously in terms of my back is a luxury I cannot afford—no matter how innocuous the circumstances may seem. I have to be continuously mindful of my body mechanics. Under the influence of acute intense pain, the idea of not using narcotics can still seem completely foreign to me. Of course there are circumstances under which taking opioids for acute or post-surgical pain is a true medical necessity. Even still, in such scenarios, recovering addicts have special risks and responsibilities that require coordinated planning and precautions, including working closely with one's doctor(s), sponsor, and significant others.

My experience continues to teach me that I can stay solution-oriented and in recovery: if I do not act on impulse and immediately buy into whatever bullshit my automatic thoughts and self-talk may be trying to sell me; if I allow myself to embrace my feelings even when I don't want to, to truly feel them whether they are positive or painful; and if I can stay fundamentally present-centered and open to the full range of possibilities. Many of those possibilities, such as walking through this injury without the aid of opioids, are beyond my conscious awareness at any given moment in time. It is only by letting each moment blossom and take its own course that I have access to its unique opportunities for learning, growing, and healing.

chapter sixteen

[PERSONALITY CHALLENGES AND] SPIRITUAL PRINCIPLES

"Fill your bowl to the rim and it will spill.
Keep sharpening your knife and it will blunt."

TAO TE CHING, VERSE 9

About four months after I returned to Tucson following my stint in treatment at Las Vegas Recovery Center, seemingly out of the blue my sponsor Phil told me, "You're gonna end up working in Las Vegas (for LVRC)." Taken by surprise I remarked, "What the hell are you talking about?" He said that he just had a strong feeling it would happen. I respectfully disagreed, suggesting that, although the idea had it charms, it was exceedingly unlikely, especially given that I was in the process of negotiating the surrender of my state Social Work license. Subsequently, every three months or so, during one of our regular conversations, Phil would spontaneously ask, "They got a job for you in Vegas yet?" His certainty, divorced from reality as it appeared to be, was comical, yet curious.

The first time I returned to Las Vegas came in the spring of 2008. I had been in recovery for eighteen months, and drove the seven hours from Tucson to attend an LVRC alumni reunion gathering. It warmed my heart to see the staff, some of the folks with whom I had been in treatment, and alumni from "graduating classes" before and after mine. It was there that I met Nancy Schenck, the Executive Editor of Central Recovery Press (CRP), a new publishing company specializing in addiction treatment, recovery, and behavioral healthcare-related topics. CRP is part of Central Recovery, the parent company of LVRC.

Nancy, who has been in recovery herself since 1982, and I hit it off immediately, talking at length about recovery and Central Recovery Press—in particular about an upcoming book project on the therapeutic value of pets in the recovery process. This book would present first-person accounts by recovering addicts of the hope and healing they derived from their pets, and CRP was currently looking for people to contribute stories. One thing led to another, and when *Tails of Recovery: Addicts and the Pets That Love Them* was published in the spring of 2009, it contained two stories I had written pertaining to my younger daughter's dog and my cat respectively (using pseudonyms to err on the side of protecting the anonymity of my daughters).

In October of 2008, shortly before my divorce became final, Nancy called to tell me that CRP had grown to the point where they were looking to add a full-time staff writer position, and invited me to apply. The ideal candidate was someone with the requisite writing skills (no shit), was in recovery, and had a behavioral health background. Everything fell into place as if it was meant to happen exactly as it did. It was an offer I couldn't refuse—that is, unless I wanted to risk giving the universe my middle finger. With considerable amusement I called Phil to say, "Guess what?"

About six months after I moved to Las Vegas, Phil and I agreed that it would serve me best to transition to a local sponsor. By this time I was well-established in my twelve-step program in Vegas—I had a service position in my home group and attended multiple meetings per week. I had become acquainted with many local fellowship members, a handful of which I viewed as having the breadth and depth of recovery I was looking for in a sponsor (Phil was a tough act to follow). Jimmy happened to be a long-time friend of Phil's, who at that time had been in recovery for twenty-four years. He carried himself with an unassuming aura of integrity and quiet, but unmistakable spirituality.

In twelve-step recovery we usually engage in a structured process of "working" the steps with a sponsor as part of learning about each step and how they relate to recovery in detail, en route to actively applying the principles of the steps in our lives on a day-to-day basis. I had completed Steps One through Five with Phil prior to moving from Tucson, and he, Jimmy, and I came up with a novel way for me to complete Step Six and transition to Jimmy for sponsorship. Like Phil and I, Jimmy was a passionate long-term aficionado of the Grateful Dead, and the then current post-Jerry Garcia incarnation of the band, The Dead, was playing in Los Angeles a few weeks hence. Phil flew up to Vegas from Tucson and the three of us drove to LA for the concert.

We went over my Sixth Step at great length on the drive there, with Phil and Jimmy double-teaming me with their complementary styles. Jimmy quickly picked up on my tendency to get stuck in my head and intellectualize my feelings. He reflected this observation directly, but with gentleness and compassion. We had a great time at the concert, reveling in music we adored and the shared experience of it. On the drive back to Vegas the next day, Jimmy formally became my sponsor. All was well, really well, and then my car died on the side of Interstate 15 in the Mojave Desert ninety miles south of Vegas in the middle of fucking nowhere—reminding me once again how quickly so much can change.

The only specific promise my twelve-step program makes is "freedom from active addiction." But since recovery is much more than mere abstinence, once liberated from the straightjacket of the obsession and compulsion to use, the locus of attention expands to include in-depth examination of the content of one's character and its relationship to quality of life considerations. In Step Six of the Twelve Steps, the primary tasks are to identify the specific aspects of one's personality that get in the way of learning, growing, and healing, and become ready to relinquish them. The Sixth Step is about developing conscious awareness of—in the parlance of twelve-step recovery—the "defects of character" that pose internal obstacles to ongoing recovery, the kind of person we want to be, and the kind of life we want to live. Step Six fits together hand-in-glove with Step Seven, which is about drawing on a burgeoning sense of spirituality as a resource to help remove those character defects or "shortcomings," or at minimum, reduce their influence in our lives.

Character defects, as ominous and malignant as the term may sound, are merely personality traits—attributes, reactions, and attitudes—that create problems for us in coping with life as it is. They tend to emerge and become more prominent in response to stress, and emotional and physical pain. It may be more helpful to view them as character challenges. In fact, everyone, whether they struggle with addiction or chronic pain, or any other serious condition, or not, has certain personality challenges that can be problematic. We are really talking about basic human qualities and the ways of relating to oneself, to others, and to the world—that have become exaggerated and distorted, contributing to imbalance and creating additional suffering for us and those around us—as a result of the obsessive thinking, compulsive behaving, and self-centered attitudes that have become hardwired in the disease of addiction and/or the crucible of chronic pain.

Personality is a psychological construct consisting of a set of characteristics that make a person uniquely who he or she is. Our personality impacts our thoughts, emotions, motivations, attitudes, and behaviors. As described in the *DSM*, personality traits are consistent and lasting patterns of perceiving and relating to oneself and one's environment that are displayed in a wide range of social and personal contexts. Personality traits can be thought of as relatively stable characteristics that sway individuals to behave in certain ways. Everyone has a variety of different personality traits, some are adaptive; others are problematic. The totality of each person's unique personality coalesces from the combination and interaction of their various traits.

One of the best-known theories of personality is Erik Erikson's model of psychosocial development. Like Freud, Erikson believed that personality develops in a series of stages. However, unlike Freud's theory of psychosexual stages, which posits that adult personality is explicitly dependent upon early childhood experiences and largely determined by age five, Erikson's approach highlights the impact of family and social interactions on personality development through eight stages across the entire lifespan, from infancy to old age.

According to Erikson, our sense of self is constantly evolving due to new experiences and information we acquire through interactions with others, and a coherent sense of self is promoted through experiences of competence, while an incomplete sense of self and feelings of inadequacy result from developmental needs that go unmet and conflicts that remain unresolved. A sense of inadequacy and the need to avoid the distress it causes is a common contributing factor in the genesis of addiction, as well as one of its concomitant effects. I've described at length how this dynamic played out for me.

Consistent with Erik Erikson's view, the past is often present in our reactions to people and situations, tinting the lenses through which we see with residue from earlier in life, based on experiences growing up in our families of origin and from previous stages of psychosocial development. Many reactions are unconscious and automatic, like a reflex. When a doctor checks your reflexes, he or she taps you just below the knee with that special rubber hammer, and if your reflexes are working well, your foot jumps up. You don't have to think about it, it just happens . . . instantly.

Personality challenges breed reactions that are especially prone to reflex. In childhood, these reactions often served the purposes of self-protection and bolstering self-image. Come adulthood most have outlived any usefulness they had and now only interfere with the ability to respond skillfully to the vicissitudes of life. Reactions driven by personality challenges are impulsive and immediate. It is frequently not how the person intended to act, and rarely how they wanted to act. Such reactions are consistently self-defeating, and destructive, usually making the situation, and how everyone involved feels about it, worse.

The more my reactions occur automatically, under the influence of my personality challenges, the more likely they are to cause suffering for myself and those around me. And I always feel guilty about it. This is why, of the Twelve Steps, Steps Six and Seven are among my favorites. The Sixth Step gives me a mechanism to identify the specific forms that my personality challenges assume so that I can become more aware of them, exercise greater conscious choice with regard to acting on them, and begin the process of letting them go. The Seventh Step provides steps (pun intended) I can take to ameliorate these challenges and the impulses they feed that lead me to reflexively act like an asshole, allowing me to be a better person by responding to circumstances in ways that are much more mindful, proportionate, and balanced.

As illustrated in preceding chapters, my personality challenges take a range of forms, including rapid frustration and escalation to anger, impatience, intolerance, arrogance, perfectionism, self-centeredness, rebelliousness, being controlling, and being judgmental. I can also be savagely sarcastic, hyper-competitive, stubborn, insecure, self-righteous, overly-critical, self-pitying, resentful, overly-analytical, demanding, defensive, inclined toward procrastination, and prone to schadenfreude (those are the highlights). Steps Six and Seven give me the gift of not having to go on autopilot mode and act out on these character challenges in reaction to my emotional or physical pain.

As I described using the pressure cooker analogy, uncomfortable and painful feelings always find a path to expression, and if we do not acknowledge these feelings consciously, by allowing ourselves to feel them and talk about them, they come out indirectly via our reactions, attitudes, and behavior. Personality challenges often rear their heads as if by reflex in emotionally charged situations that bring up difficult, threatening feelings. For example, arrogance—believing oneself to be better than others—emerges in reaction to feeling insecure/believing oneself to be less than others. Similarly, defensiveness is a personality challenge that occurs when people feel as if they are under some sort of emotional attack. Anger and aggression are shortcomings that frequently take place in reaction to feelings of upset, hurt, or fear. Acting out on personality challenges is frequently a signal that you are experiencing intense feelings.

Being judgmental about a quality in others is a personality challenge that frequently emerges when there is unconscious discomfort with the same quality in oneself. Often, when people focus on others in negative and judgmental ways, the defense mechanism of projection is in operation. Projection occurs when we attribute to other people the unacceptable thoughts, feelings, and qualities that we have but are unable to consciously acknowledge because they don't fit with our self-image and are too uncomfortable or painful. We see in others what we cannot see in ourselves. It's always easier and more comfortable to focus on others than it is to focus on oneself. In the twelve-step programs, there is a saying that suggests projection is hard at work: "If you spot it (in others), you got it (in yourself)." For example, I often react with judgment and intolerance when a speaker is long-winded; yet I am frequently long-winded myself.

Personality challenges are a normal and natural part of being human, and exist on a continuum for every person—from very little of a prickly personality trait to a truckload of it. Even people who are models of mental and emotional health can display some degree of impatience, intolerance, judgmentalness, insecurity, defensiveness, disproportionate frustration or anger, self-centeredness, etc. from time to time.

The constitutional make-up of addicts combines with their experiences before and during active addiction to amplify their susceptibility to personality challenges. Addicts are likely to have more personality challenges, and are more likely to act out on them, as well as to evince more intense and problematic forms of them. Those who struggle with chronic pain or any serious chronic condition that generates enduring physical and emotional pain are also more likely to have more personality challenges and act out on them more frequently.

Interestingly, quite a few personality traits are healthy and adaptive up to a point—until they cross a threshold, become imbalanced, and turn into challenges. They become problematic or "defective" whenever they precipitate reactions, in thinking, feeling, and/or behaving that are obsessive, compulsive, extreme or disproportionate to the situation, and cause suffering for oneself and/or others.

For instance, guilt is a form of emotional distress or discomfort that occurs naturally when we believe that we've made a mistake, committed some wrong, or failed in an obligation. Guilt can be healthy and helpful in that it's a signal that we have violated our own values or a more universal ethical-moral code, harmed someone, or otherwise acted inappropriately. Guilt helps keep people honest and self-aware in ways that contribute to emotional balance. In contrast, guilt becomes a personality challenge when we assume more than our fair share of responsibility for problems or mistakes, or believe that it's somehow our fault when things go wrong for which we are not responsible.

Guilt becomes unhealthy and creates unnecessary suffering for me when my self-blame is blown out of proportion, and I use it to beat myself up. For many addicts, it is easy to fall into a pattern of guilt-driven self-blame: for being an addict; for the consequences related to one's active addiction, including damage to relationships, health, and finances; for not being able to get a good-enough job; for not having a better living situation; for not being farther along in recovery; etc.

Competitiveness can be a personality challenge, but in and of itself, being competitive is not a problem nor does it create problems. Competitiveness can be a positive quality, based on the normal, natural, and healthy desire to do well and perform at a high level in specific activities or in general. Being competitive can help motivate people put forth the effort and dedication needed to perform well and be successful in many important life areas, including school and work.

Competitiveness becomes maladaptive and creates suffering when the need to be "better than" others or "the best" becomes a priority that overrides all others. It can become out of balance to the point where virtually everything is viewed as a competition that *must be* won, adversely affecting how we treat ourselves and others, and interfering with relationships and other priorities. In general, I'm nowhere near as competitive as I once was; however, sports can still ignite a regression to a mindset of overbearing competitiveness. Moreover, when it comes to athletic pursuits, I'm competing with the ironclad expectations I place on my own performance, in addition to whatever individual or team I may be playing against.

At this point in my life, the competition with my own expectations is more heated than that with any external opponent. I've learned how to lose to others graciously and with acceptance—as long as I perform within the ballpark of my expectations. When my performance fails to measure up to these exacting self-imposed standards, I wrestle with being painfully aggrieved—filled with frustration, anger, and inadequacy—and it can be "fugly" (as in fucking ugly). Although the intensity of these emotions and the reactions they fuel dissipate much more quickly than they used to, in the meantime they can still create suffering for me and those closest to me.

My competiveness dovetails with another of my personality challenges: perfectionism. Perfectionism is a common response to emotional pain. The need to be perfect permits no room for mistakes or vulnerability. My perfectionism is among my oldest comrades, following me around like a shadow, providing an inexhaustible source of kindling for self-criticism. Dynamically, perfectionism is the flipside of not believing oneself to be "good enough." It is another striking example of the defense mechanism of reaction formation, wherein the thoughts, feelings, and attitudes expressed are the opposite of those actually held—which are so distressing that they are sequestered outside of conscious awareness. If I'm perfect, I can banish all thoughts and feelings of inadequacy.

Too bad perfection is an illusory objective and the epitome of an unrealistic expectation. Perfectionism inevitably rebounds upon itself, reinforcing the belief that who I am is not good enough. It's like trying to hold onto water—I may achieve it for a few moments, but it's impossible to maintain. The harder I try to grasp it, the more completely it slips through my fingers. I have vivid memories of this dynamic at work when sharpening my pencil in elementary school. The need to achieve the perfect point led me to continue to sharpen the pencil past the point where it was already more than good enough—until it broke . . . repeatedly. I might go through this self-defeating exercise four or five times before the pencil point was either satisfactory or I gave in, feeling as though I couldn't get it right. With each successive iteration of this self-induced torment my suffering escalated. Under the influence of perfectionism, the perfect is the sworn enemy of the good enough.

During the summer when I was eleven, we visited friends of my parents who had rented a house on the beach in Mattituck on the north fork of eastern Long Island. While swimming in the shallow waveless water of Long Island Sound, I spied several small pufferfish darting about and determined that I was going to catch one—with my bare hands. When I announced this to my parents and their friends, they all chuckled, assuring me I was being unrealistic and that it would never happen. I spent the next three hours doggedly pursuing my elusive prize. It was more frustrating than fun but after coming very close a few times, I caught one. Cupping it in my hands with a feeling that combined relief and elated accomplishment, I walked up the beach wearing a triumphant smile, to show the adults who were appropriately chastened and impressed. In that moment, everything was perfect, even me. Of course, it couldn't last, though I wasn't willing to let it go. I held onto to it tightly, attempting to bring the pufferfish home in a bucket of water from the Sound. It died later that day.

Perfectionism frequently arises when significant people from early in our lives impose unrealistic expectations on us and we internalize them, effectively taking on those same expectations and making them our own. Mistakes become unacceptable and no matter what we do, it is never good enough. It has to be fucking perfect. Phil described such negative self-perceptions as "the lies that other people have told us about ourselves," and that their need to criticize or put others down was a function of their own emotional baggage. It was "their bag of rocks." Whenever I buy into and start to believe the lies that other people have told me about me, they become my bag of rocks. Bearing the burden of its weight and bulk, I carry it with me wherever I go.

Those of us who toil under the yoke of perfectionism do whatever we can to try to feel good enough about ourselves, while the perception that we are somehow falling short and there is always more we could have or should have done gnaws at us. The implications of this psychological schema were clarified for me, when, in my fourth year of recovery I heard my dear friend Nancy (who had twenty-eight years in recovery at that time) share that painting oneself with broad-brush negative labels based on feelings of inadequacy is a form of self-mutilation, no less injurious than cutting oneself.

The other aspect of the Sixth Step involves becoming ready to let go of our identified personality challenges. The process of letting go of the old and unhealthy is at the heart of moving from the darkness of active addiction into the light of recovery. Consistent with Taoist and Buddhist approaches, letting go begins when I become consciously aware of how I create suffering for myself and others. The letting go of personality challenges is actually a continuation of the process that occurred in each of the previous steps. It is the process of surrendering the things that separate me from others so I can move beyond what no longer works:

- In Step One, I let go of the belief that I was not an addict; I let go of using and thinking that I could control it and that my life was okay as it was.

- In Step Two, I let go of the belief that I could recover from my addiction without the help of powers beyond myself.

- In Step Three, I began to let go of the need to control other people and situations, as well as to be "right," by establishing a conscious connection to that which is beyond myself.

- In Steps Four and Five, I let go of the dishonesty and secrets that I had held onto and guarded closely for so many years, and began to shed some of the shame that went with them.

Many people naturally act out on the problematic features of their personality in situations that are stressful, uncomfortable, or painful because that is what they have always done. Even if they've made a commitment to themselves and others that they won't act that way any more, like a reflex reaction it happens automatically, and continues to happen. While conscious awareness is extremely important, knowing that something isn't working is not enough to change behavior. If the awareness that specific reactions and attitudes create serious problems was all that was necessary, changing them would be a hell of a lot easier. The only way to make those kinds of positive and healthy life changes is to act differently. If I want different results, I have to do things differently.

The work of Steps Six and Seven is designed to counteract the habitual impulses people have to act out on their personality challenges. And just because someone has multiple years of recovery doesn't mean that they are beyond acting in ways that cause suffering for themselves and others. It can be deceptively easy to fall back into operating on autopilot, where the re-emergence of those problematic aspects of personality just sort of happens.

The quality of someone's recovery is evident in his or her actions, rather than in his or her words. This is especially true with regard to the work people have done (or not done) on their personality challenges. For example, some people are very impressive in twelve-step meetings, speaking about spiritual principles in ways that are inspiring and seem inspired. But, when the meeting is over, they might engage in petty gossip, pass judgment on others, or display arrogance, among other common shortcomings. As Phil would say, "Inside meetings they're a supernova, but outside they're a Chevy Nova."

Spirituality has always been a fundamental component of twelve-step philosophy and practice. Scientific research has demonstrated that higher levels of spirituality and involvement in spiritual practices are linked with measurable improvements in specific quality of life areas. There is a positive correlation between the practice of Step Eleven (with its emphasis on meditation and prayer) and generally higher spirituality levels among twelve-step program members and life satisfaction, among other outcomes. Moreover, other aspects of spirituality, including a sense of purpose, gratitude, and forgiveness,[24, 25] as well as the belief in a higher power were correlated with a higher quality of recovery as measured by the degree of inner peace, degree of personal growth, and ratings of relationships.[26]

Step Seven involves identifying the specific spiritual principles that represent the opposites of our personality challenges. As noted previously, accepting our feelings and allowing ourselves to feel them takes less energy than avoiding, suppressing, or displacing them by acting out on the personality challenges they drive. Genuine acceptance of feelings frees up energy to practice spiritual principles in response to whatever life throws at us. The dialectical dynamics of acceptance and change are active in the Seventh Step. The work combines the acceptance of my feelings with improving conscious contact with spiritual principles—through practice applying them to dislodge my personality challenges. The most effective path to personality renovation is to practice the spiritual opposites of one's personality challenges.

Personality challenges and the spiritual principles that oppose them cannot operate at the same time. If the treatment for the disease of addiction is actively working a program of recovery (often in combination with some level of formal professional treatment), the treatment for one's personality challenges is the active application of spiritual principles. The antidote for my inclination to judge others is compassion—for others and for myself. The antidote for my arrogance is humility. The antidote for my resentment—old anger kept alive by the reliving of past perceived injustices in my mind—is forgiveness.

The antidote for my anger is acceptance. My twelve-step literature describes anger as my reaction to and denial of the present. Acceptance is about being okay with things as they are in the here and now. At first, I didn't understand the link between anger and denial. It took me a while to appreciate that they are simply different stops on the same mental-emotional rail line. Denial is a function of the inability to accept reality as it is. Anger is a more conscious form of denial that reflects my refusal, my unwillingness to accept reality.

Anger is my narcissistic denunciation of reality that I don't like because circumstances or people aren't how I want them to be or think they should be. This happens in bowling, when I throw what appears to be a perfect strike ball that crushes the pocket at the ideal angle of entry, blowing up all the pins—except for the number ten pin (the pin of Satan for right-handed bowlers the world over), which somehow remains completely untouched and stands there taunting me. How dare that muthafuckingpieceofshit pin defy my will and not fall down with the rest of them like it was supposed to—damn it! Whenever I'm unable to accept the reality I'm presented with, my anger ignites and suffering commences.

Here too, the convergence between twelve-step recovery, Buddhism, and Western psychotherapy is discernible. In Buddhism, anger, resentment, and general ill-will are recognized as fundamental obstacles to spiritual development. A common Buddhist technique for resolving anger is the use of active contemplation or meditation using *metta*—loving-kindness and compassion, initially directed inward toward oneself, and then outward to others, including the objects of our anger. It is virtually impossible for loving kindness and/or compassion and anger to be felt simultaneously.

Albert Ellis, the psychologist who developed Rational Emotive Behavior Therapy (REBT), was a central figure in the emergence of cognitive behaviorally-oriented forms of psychotherapy, and is sometimes considered the godfather of cognitive behavioral therapy (CBT). Ellis described the cognitive behavioral technique known as "emotional training" in strikingly similar terms. In emotional training, a person endeavors to replace his or her hostile feelings toward someone with positive feelings by recalling pleasant experiences associated with that individual along with the related feelings, and having those positive feelings supplant the anger.

Consciously reframing situations that can evoke my impulsive over-the-top reactions is another way to displace my personality challenges with spiritual principles. As mentioned before, all our experiences have a certain structure that includes the context (where we are, who we're with, what's happening around us), our expectations, and the interpretations or meanings we assign to it. Whenever there are changes to that structure, it causes changes in the subjective experience. Reframing is a communication technique that has its origins in the work of Milton Erickson, and is utilized in Neuro-linguistic Programming (NLP), among other psychotherapeutic models. Reframing consists of adjusting how we view a situation; looking at it from another perspective, with the result that it evokes a different meaning and new possibilities, translating to modified, usually more balanced, thoughts, feelings, and behavioral responses.

For example, being stuck in traffic is naturally frustrating. Many people, especially when confronted by encroaching time constraints, (and who among us isn't regularly subjected to time constraints) struggle in this scenario as anger rises and tempers flare. My personality challenges of impatience, rapid frustration, and escalation to anger are summoned to the fore, with my habitual behavioral reaction—the impulse to act out on them by cursing (perhaps hard to believe) loudly and repeatedly—in hot pursuit.

I can utilize a handful of different recovery-related skills to adjust my response, including the Serenity Prayer, which modifies my perspective by framing the situation as being beyond my control, thereby shifting my attention toward acceptance strategies. However, my preferred self-intervention is a reframe that views the traffic as a message from that which is beyond me to mindfully slow myself down, and use the experience as an opportunity to practice the spiritual principles of patience, tolerance, and acceptance. Whenever I can do this, my conscious contact with these spiritual principles crowds out the relevant personality challenges, freeing me from their grip. It's as if my internal operating system has been upgraded with new, better functioning software. My breathing slows and deepens; the space between stimulus and response (so wonderfully described by Viktor Frankl) widens, and my conscious attention returns to the here and now.

One of the secondary gains of this process is that I have progressively become a more mindful, easygoing, and safe driver. I used to always be in a hurry, anxious to get to wherever I was going, even when there was plenty of time to reach my intended destination. When I implement the values of slowing down and paying attention with intention, the effects carry over to all areas of my life, including my driving. When approaching an intersection with a yellow light, I'm now more likely to slow down and prepare to stop than to accelerate in an attempt to beat the light before it turns red. And even more improbable to me, I can usually wait without worry or frustration until the light turns green. Though I am still susceptible to occasional bouts of (as a friend refers to it) "vehicular Tourettes"—sudden outbursts of profanity in reaction to road conditions or other drivers—they have become much fewer and farther between.

While relapse into drug use is not part of my story (just for today), I do have periodic relapses of acting out on my personality challenges, including the need to control and to "be right." Fortunately, the more I practice applying the spiritual principles of my program of recovery from addiction and chronic pain, the quicker I become consciously aware that I'm caught up in a familiar unhealthy and unhelpful vortex. I can then make a conscious decision about how I want to act, rather than react unconsciously based on well worn reflexive patterns. It's like realizing (awareness) that the plane I'm piloting is nose-diving toward a crash and then using the skills I've acquired to pull out of that dive (action). With practice, I act out on my personality challenges less often, and when I do act out on them, my actions are less severe and create less suffering for me and those I care about. And progressively I develop the capacity to be kinder and gentler with everyone, even me.

It's useful to clarify that personality challenges may never be totally removed in the sense that they disappear altogether. Through awareness and action, it is possible to behave differently, downsizing the prevalence, intensity, and influence of these challenges so that they create fewer problems. As their sharp edges are chipped away and their rough spots sanded down, their power over me and my behavior decreases.

The diligent practicing of spiritual principles gradually and progressively turns personality challenges from huge boulders that obstruct one's path into small smooth stones that can be sidestepped or picked up and tossed aside. However, it's still easy to trip over even small stones if I'm not paying enough conscious attention to where I'm walking in the here and now.

chapter seventeen

[ROOTS THEN WINGS]

"Sometimes we live no particular way but our own
Sometimes we visit your country and live in your home
Sometimes we ride on your horses
Sometimes we walk alone.
Sometimes the songs that we hear
Are just songs of our own.
Wake up to find out that you are the eyes of the world."

ROBERT HUNTER, *EYES OF THE WORLD*, GRATEFUL DEAD

Both my kids are wonderful in many ways. I have been blessed with children who are so much better than I ever was (my parents would gladly attest to that; they seemed genuinely disappointed when it became clear that their promise would never come to fruition; you know, "Don't worry, you'll have one just like yourself one day!"). And yet, just doing what came naturally to them, essentially what they were "supposed" to do at whatever ages they were, whether it was two, six, nine, thirteen, sixteen, etc., on occasion, they have still been excellent ads for birth control.

And then there are the complexities of being the father of daughters. When my older daughter was about sixteen, I was doing the family laundry when I came across an article of clothing that I didn't recognize. It was foreign enough to me that I took a few moments to study it in the attempt to figure out what the hell it was. It looked like it could have been an eye patch, though that seemed unlikely. With a frightening flash of "oh my fucking god" recognition, it dawned on me that I was holding my daughter's thong.

Around that time, she also started dating. I have always been a staunch advocate of gun control, so it was a bit jarring when we moved to Arizona, given its pervasive Wild West mentality and everyone-should-be-able-to-take-a-gun-pretty-much-anywhere-they-damn-well-please laws. But as I began to anticipate close encounters with prospective boyfriends, the idea of owning a gun started to make sense, and two questions arose: What caliber? And, do I turn it first on my daughters' potential suitors or keep it simple and just turn it on myself?

It was August of 2009, and my older daughter had just moved to Washington, DC. She graduated from Arizona State University in May of that year with a major in Political Science and a minor in Spanish. She had evolved into a remarkable young woman. She spent most of her senior year at ASU working in the Tempe, Arizona, office of the US congressman there, Harry Mitchell. As an unpaid intern during the fall semester, she did so well that when one of the regular staff took a temporary leave, she was hired to fill that position, and ultimately spent six months as a paid congressional staff person, writing pieces that the congressman read into the Congressional Record and providing constituent services.

Having determined that government can be a helpful part of the solution to the ills that afflict our society, she decided to pursue a career path related to government service, and was committed to continuing her formal education with a Masters in Public Administration. She had the choice of staying at ASU where she was familiar and very comfortable, or forsaking the known and seeking out much greater potential for growth and opportunity in Washington, DC, at George Washington University. To her great credit, she took the healthy risk of stepping 2,500 miles outside of her comfort zone.

Leaving everything that one knows is a tremendous challenge fraught with uncertainty, stress, anxiety, confusion, and fear, even under the most promising circumstances. It takes strength and courage to venture beyond our existing frame of reference. Most people choose to stay inside their boxes of familiarity and emotional safety out of fear of the uncertainty of the unknown. Yet, going beyond that which we already know is often the greatest generator of learning and growth.

Ambivalence is intrinsic to every momentous decision—those life-altering forks in the road that directly shape the course of our lives. Anyone who tries to convince us otherwise is either in denial or full of shit. Such choice points include getting married, buying a house, and having children, as well as relocating across considerable distances. This was certainly the case for my daughter as she moved cross-country, attempting to negotiate a completely new environment starting with finding a place to live in a large, crowded, and very expensive city. At times this was a real struggle for her. She needed a place that was convenient to school, more or less affordable, and most importantly safe. As her search lasted longer than she had hoped, she was alternately terrified, hopeful, depressed, determined, and naturally, extremely ambivalent about whether this was the right move for her.

Becoming a parent nearly twenty-two years earlier had introduced me to an entirely new level of emotional agony. In my experience, there is no greater love than that for one's children—but the other side of that coin is that here is no greater pain than to see, hear, or feel my kids in pain and to have to confront my limitations to ease it—regardless of whether their pain is physical, emotional, or a combination of the two. It is a gut-wrenching heartache. In phone calls with me, my daughter put on a generally brave face. I only learned that this was a front through conversations with my ex-wife as we tried to coordinate our efforts to be helpful. That my daughter apparently didn't feel comfortable showing me the depth of her difficulty, and knowing that I needed to respect this boundary she had set (as much as I wanted to tell her, "I know what the deal is, please get real and talk to me!") only added to my own upset and sense of helplessness.

So, it was a relief all around when she signed a lease on a studio apartment in an older building with a lobby staffed twenty-four/seven located virtually right on the GWU campus in close proximity to the State Department in the Foggy Bottom section of DC—a good, safe (relatively speaking) part of the city. My daughter and I had agreed that when she got a place, I'd fly out to help her furnish and generally set it up. I had no time available to take off from work so this meant accomplishing my mission over the course of a single weekend. Moreover, at the time, I was under serious financial stress. But what mattered most was that she needed my help and I needed to be there for her in this way. As Phil, my original sponsor from Tucson taught me, it's about suiting up and showing up, no matter what. As Jimmy, my current sponsor emphasized, regardless of the challenges, to be able to be there for my daughter in whatever way I could, would be a great blessing for me, as well as for her.

My whirlwind weekend involved over fifteen hours traveling to and from DC in exchange for forty-four hours on the ground there. By the time I made it to my daughter's place it was 1:00 a.m. on Saturday. After an essentially sleepless night on her floor, I spent the next two days driving a big-ass U-Haul truck in world-class traffic throughout the District, northern Virginia, and southern Maryland, to pick up furniture so we could haul it up to her fourth floor apartment.

Our first order of business was to pick up a bed she was buying through Craigslist from a family in McLean, Virginia. The two largest pieces she needed were a sofa and a queen-size bed. Just because she's all of 5'3" and 120 pounds doesn't mean she didn't require a queen-size bed (the denial inherent in being the father of daughters generally protects me from considering the possibility of her sharing it). It just so happened that the sellers were also looking to unload their living room sofa that my daughter readily agreed to purchase with her own money.

Initially, it seemed like a fortuitous twist of fate that the sofa she needed appeared so conveniently. However, I quickly started to have a nagging sense that this sofa might well be too big to get into her apartment. It was really nice, but long and wide and extremely deep—the kind that can be slept on easily and comfortably, and so cushy you could lose a small child in it. On the drive back to DC, my concern that the sofa was just too damn big forced its way to conscious expression, taking up more and more space in my head. I started to kick myself in the ass for not being more aware of this, and shared my concern with my daughter. At best, it would just barely fit, and I began to hope against hope for this outcome.

Arriving back at her building, the person staffing the front desk directed us to the service elevator, accessible only through the back of the building. We carefully maneuvered the U-Haul through the narrow back alley, parked, and began to check out the route between the truck and her apartment. It was ridiculously circuitous: down a long steep set of concrete stairs; making a ninety-degree turn at the bottom into the basement, negotiating two more tight turns in a narrow hallway with a ceiling made considerably lower by hanging pipes and ductwork, all just to get to the so-called "service" elevator. This elevator was approximately five to six feet long, three to four feet wide, and perhaps seven feet high. It appeared to be the exact same size as the building's passenger elevator, the only difference being the heavy duty moving-type blankets covering the walls. While this padding protected the elevator from damage, it effectively made it even smaller. My heart sank, as I knew we were completely screwed; even if we could get the sofa to the elevator, there was no way in hell it was going to fit.

That notwithstanding, I was bound and determined to do everything I could to try. If there was any way possible to make it work, I would find it.

If it was a physical impossibility, I would have to confirm it with absolute certainty. This wasn't a function of denial. It was a need to problem-solve to the best of my ability for my daughter. She had spent a big chunk of her limited funds on that sofa and I was not in a position where I could replace them. I felt guilty that I hadn't voiced my concerns about the sofa's size in a timely way, and dammit she needed a sofa. And this was the only opportunity to fulfill this need during my brief stay, after which her opportunities to take care of this would be very limited.

I enlisted the building maintenance guy to help me lug the Olympic-size sofa through the bowels of the building in several fruitless, increasingly frustrating, and sweat-soaked attempts to find a successful route to my daughter's apartment. All the while, my back was under tremendous duress and even with a good support belt, my lumbar spine was shrieking. But I didn't hear it. I couldn't listen to it. I was on a mission. We got the sofa all the way to the service elevator and tried every possible way we could think of, using multiple angles of approach, but it just wouldn't fit. My daughter looked like she was close to crying, and I was crestfallen.

As I mentioned earlier, the Serenity Prayer may be the simplest, yet most elegant coping device ever devised. Most every situation can be placed in one of two categories: those I can change in some way, shape, or form; and those that are beyond my capacity to influence or change. The more I practice applying this spiritual template in real life circumstances as they smack me upside the head, the better at it I get.

I chose to focus on the second part of the Serenity Prayer, in this case trying to change things that I hoped I could. Not ready in that moment, to accept what a part of me knew to be inevitable, we wrestled the sofa back through the winding, narrow basement hallway, up the long steep concrete stairs, put it back in the truck and drove it around to the building's main entrance. I pleaded for and received reticent permission from the front desk staff to bring the sofa in through the main lobby with its higher ceilings and greater room to maneuver, praying silently that the sofa would somehow fit into the passenger elevator.

We again tried every conceivable way to get that upholstered monstrosity into the elevator, attempting to bend the laws of physics during an epic struggle. Although we came closer to fitting it in, the sofa's combination of length, width, and depth simply made it too fucking big.

Drained and exhausted, I came to the place where I had no alternative but to admit defeat and accept that which I could not change. The only thing we could do at that point was to carry the sofa back to the truck, drive it around the back of the building again, and leave it by the dumpster. Perhaps someone else would have the space for it. My daughter and I were both devastated.

My only solace was that I knew with certainty I'd done everything I could, and that my daughter had witnessed it in all its physical, emotional, and sweat-soaked intensity. I could strive for acceptance without second guessing whether there was another way, maybe . . . somehow . . . if only . . . nope . . . no fucking way. Part of my learning, growing, and healing is the awareness that when I encounter "things" I cannot change, and therefore need to accept, there remains one thing I always have the ability to change: how I respond to such situations.

Trying to change the things I can't only makes the situation, whatever it might be, worse. It's like spitting into a headwind—it gets blown back on me and those closest to me. In addition to putting the Serenity Prayer into action, I needed to apply Step One and surrender to the reality of the situation and accept my powerlessness over it (fuck!).

It put a serious damper on the emotional tone of the afternoon, but only temporarily. My daughter and I wore the residual frustration, sadness, and upset like a saturated sweatshirt for a couple of hours until it had outlived any usefulness and we took it off to focus on the remaining work of the day. This included returning the U-Haul to one of the more dangerous parts of the District, taking the car I had rented at the airport to an IKEA in College Park, Maryland, and getting as many of the remaining furnishings she needed as we could afford and fit into the car.

On the return trip to her apartment we found ourselves in the middle of a many-miles-long traffic jam that seemed to stretch to the horizon. We were worn so thin at that point. In order to turn the rising feelings of helplessness (as if I hadn't already experienced enough of that for one day) and rage down to a dull roar, we decided to take a resourceful detour, getting off Interstate 495 much earlier than planned, and slowly but progressively making our way diagonally across most of DC to get back to my daughter's building.

Her place was an easy fifteen minute walk to the Lincoln Memorial. That night, we went down to the monuments and spent time with Lincoln, the Reflecting Pool, the World War II Monument, and the Washington Monument. They were absolutely spectacular, even magical, bathed in light and the warm moist summer air. It was one of those peak experiences that, by virtue of their majesty, are immediately seared into memory.

Sometime after 11:00 p.m., we wandered into a TGI Fridays for some late night sustenance. I watched as my daughter ordered a frozen margarita the size of a small bird bath. After the travels and travails of our nearly eighteen-hour day, the stress and strain on my loudly barking back, and worn down still further by the heat and humidity of early August in DC, that margarita looked like heaven on earth.

For a brief moment, everything else faded into the background as the glistening drink seemed to double in size. This was not about "white-knuckling" through my attraction to the masterpiece of twenty-first century bartending perched oh-so-close, sitting on my hands to avoid the impulse to gulp some of hers or order one of my own. That might be abstinence, but it sure as hell is not recovery.

Understanding the differences between thoughts, emotions, and behaviors is fundamental to recovery. The ability to make conscious, healthy decisions about how I want to act in life depends on understanding these differences. Many people confuse how they feel with how they act. They have little conscious awareness that their feelings are separate from their behavior, and believe that they *have* to act the way they feel. In other words, if they feel angry, they have to act aggressively—yelling, intimidating, getting physical. If they feel fearful, they have to avoid whatever it is they are fearful of. And, if they have thoughts of using or if they feel like using and have urges or cravings to use (whether fueled by pain or not), they *have* to use.

A desire to use and the ability to not use no matter what, are not mutually exclusive. In fact, they can both operate simultaneously, and even co-exist peacefully. I learned early on in my experience as a psychotherapist that articulating the vast differences between thoughts, feelings, and actions is an important part of the psychoeducation I routinely provided in my direct practice with clients, and in clinical supervision and training with staff. As distressing as certain thoughts are, as uncomfortable as some feelings might be, they can't cause harm. It is only in how we act on those thoughts and/or feelings that we create problems—for ourselves and for others. We have little choice with regard to the thoughts that come into our head and the feelings that flow from these thoughts into our heart. However, we always retain choice when it comes to our actions.

I was gifted with liberation from the obsession to use toward the end of my first six months in recovery. Since that time, thoughts about using and any desire to use have been few and far between for me. Even still, there are inevitably times when I think about using, when I feel like using, or even (especially under the influence of significant pain) when a part of me wants to use. That is completely different from actually using.

Although thoughts and feelings of using always precede actual use (even if these are less than fully conscious), there is still a continent-sized difference between having a desire to use and actually using. It's normal, natural, understandable, and okay for an addict in recovery to think about using, to feel like using, and to want to use. As Michael, a friend in my twelve-step program is fond of saying, an addict not using is in an unnatural state. However, it's not okay to use. Just because a part of me might want to use does not mean that I have to.

So, I smiled to myself while grimacing slightly at the irony that my now-of-age daughter could dive into her mega-margarita head first while I mobilized the acceptance necessary to be content to sit poolside and watch her swim. My current capacity to practice the spiritual principles of recovery—in this instance, most notably tolerance, humility, perseverance, gratitude, and of course, acceptance—is manifest precisely in such circumstances. Situations like this hold up a mirror for me to see what my recovery looks like when it's put to a more direct test. Recovery includes being okay with not being able to have what I may want when I want it. That doesn't mean I have to like it! I simply need to be able to accept it and know how to be fundamentally okay with it.

The second day of my all-too-brief visit was much less intense and emotionally draining. We spent it shopping for groceries and housewares locally and assembling all the stuff we bought at IKEA (another exercise in patience and tolerance). When I arrived in DC, my daughter's place was basically an empty room, and by the time I left, it was pretty much (with the exception of a fucking sofa) a home. My daughter was extremely appreciative as we parted, hugging me with feeling. There are precious few experiences I treasure more than sharing such moments with my kids—especially as they have grown so rapidly toward adulthood. Those moments have become even more special since their mother and I divorced.

My professional background increased my appreciation that my primary role as a parent is to nurture my kids to grow roots, followed by wings: roots for a solid, stable, and safe foundation, and wings for them to individuate and become their own person, taking off from the runway of that secure base, and flying toward the future of their choosing, while hopefully maintaining a positive connection to their foundation and returning to visit on occasion. This process of separation-individuation is a beautiful, natural, and essential part of the circle of life.

But, as with all meaningful growth-enhancing experiences, there is an element of loss, with its concomitant feelings of ambivalence and sadness, and the need to mourn. Recovery is also a process of developing roots, then wings. Recovery also means experiencing and mourning the loss of parts of our lives and ourselves that no longer work for us, that interfere with our ongoing learning, growing, and healing. There is no growth without some loss—like the natural maturation process of snakes, people shed the skins that no longer fit them and meet their evolving needs. I have to be rooted well enough in the awareness and skills I need to not use no matter what, in order to take flight and make continued progress toward spiritual centeredness, self-acceptance, and self-actualization.

As I arrived at Reagan National Airport for the return flight home to Vegas, I felt blessed and grateful, yet found myself tearing up and sobbing silently. I sat down on the concrete steps leading to the terminal, and started crying loudly, making no effort to hide it as passersby gave me strange, uncomfortable glances. All I knew in that moment was that I needed to be present-centered with these feelings wherever they needed to take me, to simply be with them and ride their wave.

To my surprise, I had no real impulse to suppress this process. Although I was sitting in front of the main entrance to a busy terminal at a major international airport, I tuned out all the outside sights and sounds and focused on reducing the internal static. As I tuned in to the frequency of my emotions, I became conscious that my tears were of both joy and sadness: joy for this extraordinary visit; for a daughter who had grown wings and was creating her own way in the world; for the great gift of being there with and for her, and also of sadness for having to leave so soon; for her being so far away geographically; for not being able to do more; and perhaps, for not being able to *be* more. The brutal and the beautiful blended into the bittersweet.

chapter eighteen

[SPIRITUAL AWAKENINGS COME]
IN MANY DIFFERENT COLORS

"Small wheel turn by the fire and rod
Big wheel turn by the grace of God
Every time that wheel turn 'round
Bound to cover just a little more ground."
ROBERT HUNTER, *THE WHEEL*, GRATEFUL DEAD

One of the core characteristics that makes people vulnerable to addiction, and is amplified as a consequence of it, is a sense of internal emptiness—a pervasive feeling of being empty, hollow, and missing something. The specific manifestations of addiction—be it substances or activities (or both)—represent an attempt to fill this emptiness from the outside. External things such as substances, activities, material objects, jobs, money, or people, may fill this hole, but only temporarily. Growing up, even before I ever used a mind- or mood-altering substance, I recall feeling more whole, more fulfilled, in effect happier, when I received a present I wanted or went shopping and bought something that I desired. I also remember that those elevated feelings were short-lived.

Those who struggle with addiction routinely report a sense of spiritual emptiness. While the absence of spirituality in no way causes addiction, it is generally accepted that addiction has a spiritual component. This acknowledgment led to the incorporation of spirituality as an important ingredient in the process of recovery, and provides yet another intersection between Western psychology and psychotherapy and twelve-step recovery. Carl Jung, a Swiss psychiatrist and one-time protégé of Sigmund Freud, founded analytical psychology and pioneered the concepts of archetypes and the collective unconscious. Jung viewed addiction as a spiritual malady and addicts as frustrated spiritual seekers. He believed that the craving for altered states of consciousness reflected a spiritual thirst for wholeness, and that only those who have a spiritual awakening could successfully overcome the disease of addiction.

In 1930, Jung shared these insights with an alcoholic patient, who subsequently passed the information on to an associate of Bill Wilson, who in 1934 communicated Jung's take to the future co-founder of Alcoholics Anonymous (AA). Bill W's own process of achieving recovery was aided by what he described as a profound spiritual awakening, and when he and Dr. Bob Smith formulated the original Twelve Steps and established AA in 1935, the indispensable role of spirituality was formalized.

Recovery involves spiritual renewal, and it is built into the language of Step Twelve that, if we work the steps, we will have a "spiritual awakening." But what the hell does that mean, exactly? Many people have an image of an instantaneously life-changing event—the equivalent of being struck by a bolt of lightening or being spoken to by a burning bush (a la Moses) or some similarly dramatic and unmistakable occurrence. They may anticipate a sensational event that will forever change their lives for the better, permanently elevating them above the routine din of the daily grind, and giving them the secret to ongoing happiness.

Fortunately, happiness is not a requirement for recovery. Unfortunately, the late 1990s saw the emergence of a "happiness movement" that began to suggest and even insist that people "should" be happier. In its extreme form this message says that we have a responsibility to be happy, and that if we are not, we are doing something wrong. Consistent with this trend, social expectations have transformed normal, natural sadness and sorrow (as distinguished from clinical depression) into a depressive disorder. What used to be considered appropriate emotional reactions to loss and/or other painful life events are now frequently viewed as problematic or even pathological—necessitating counseling and/or medication with the ever-expanding repertoire of antidepressants.

In this context, sadness is something to "fight," to "not give in to," and to "get over." But what's wrong with feeling sad? The short answer is, absolutely nothing. Savoring the complete meal that is the human condition involves digging into a healthy portion of sadness when life serves it up, along with the rest of the full range of our emotions, to the best of our ability. Occasional heartburn and indigestion has a place in an overall healthy digestive process.

Expectations that we should find ways to be happy no matter what our circumstances are not only unrealistic, but also unhelpful and unhealthy. There is validity in the "law of attraction" and considerable power in positive thinking, but believing that by simply changing our thinking we can change anything and everything in our lives, including for example, our socioeconomic status, is downright delusional. Sometimes life is brutally challenging, and there is no easy way to get over, under, or around it. This notwithstanding, we always have choices. We can focus our conscious attention more on our problems or on potential solutions. That all important space between what life presents to us and how we respond to it is ours alone. We can seek to avoid our emotional and physical pain or learn how to accept what we can't change, while developing the skills to change what we can.

Happiness exists on a continuum—from overt joy and celebration to much more subtle serenity, contentment, satisfaction, and peace of mind. There are moments when I've been blessed with profound joy, those precious ever-so-brief glimpses of beauty, clarity, and just how perfect life can be. However, I cannot coerce such transcendent experiences. The harder I try to make them happen, the more they elude me. And they are always temporary. If I expect to keep them as if they were possessions, I invariably set myself up for disappointment. The most healthy and spiritual thing I can do is to recognize and appreciate these moments for what they are—as opposed to focusing on what they are not and will never be.

Spiritual awakenings don't necessarily happen the way I expect, along a timeline I prefer, or in a form obvious to me. In reality, spiritual awakenings can take many different, often subtle forms. And only when my eyes, ears, mind, and heart are fully open, am I positioned to recognize, receive, and appreciate them.

The best definition may be found in the actual experience of one's own shifts in conscious awareness. Spiritual awakenings can be as profound as a smack-upside-the-head, clear-as-a-bell recognition that all people, in fact, all living things are inextricably interconnected with one another and therefore deserve nothing less than compassion and empathy. They can also be as "ordinary" (though there's really nothing ordinary about it) as consciously tuning in to the chirping of birds or noticing with greater conscious clarity the magnificence of a sunset or how wonderful and fresh the desert smells after a monsoon rainstorm. And those awakenings can take virtually any form in between.

Each time I wake up from a modus operandi state of unconscious reflexive autopilot and become mindfully aware of my internal and external experience, there is an awakening of spirit. The term mindfulness is an interesting misnomer insofar as conscious awareness comes as much from the heart and spirit as from the mind. It was a revelation to rediscover that I have the ability to center myself in the present moment, observe my thoughts, and take note of my emotions without attachment or judgment. I have the capacity to adjust my attitude and outlook, and begin to have a better day anytime I make a conscious choice to do so. Just because I may have had a shitty day thus far doesn't mean that it has to continue in that direction.

For me, spiritual awakenings often evolve so gradually that they are almost imperceptible. In some cases, I haven't even noticed them consciously until they've been around for a while. For instance, to my astonishment, I can remain in conscious contact with gratitude in spite of feeling angry, sad, or fearful. The awareness that I can maintain an ongoing state of gratitude regardless of how I may feel was an important spiritual awakening for me. It took weeks after this process first started for me to realize that my awareness (and my behavior) had changed.

It's a spiritual awakening when I can identify the unhealthy and harmful experiences that happened to me during childhood and adolescence, while maintaining an appreciation that my parents did the best they were capable of at the time. I can love them and be extremely grateful for who they are, rather than wallow in who they were not and could never be. And I have been able to make amends to my parents and my siblings for my trespasses against them. We end every contact we have, whether by phone or in-person by saying to each other, "I love you."

As Norman Maclean wrote so beautifully in *A River Runs Through It and Other Stories,* "We can love completely without complete understanding." I apply the remarkable wisdom encapsulated in that statement to my relationship with my daughters. Understanding is helpful, but it isn't a requirement. My love for them transcends any conflicts we may have had or may have. I don't have to understand, agree with, or approve of all of their choices or actions in order to love them unconditionally.

A lot of people struggle with the idea of forgiving others whom they feel have wronged them. It's not uncommon for forgiveness to be confused with forgetting. However, they are two very different things. Forgiveness means consciously remembering and intentionally letting go. Forgiveness is a gift we give to ourselves—it's more for the person doing the forgiving than the party who is forgiven. To forgive is to cleanse oneself of pain and anger that separates us and keeps us stuck in the past. To paraphrase renowned psychologist John Friel, PhD, forgiveness is the willingness to give up all hope for a better past.

Before I began my journey of recovery, it never occurred to me to think of these as spiritual principles: patience, tolerance, acceptance, humility, empathy, compassion, loving-kindness, forgiveness, serenity, trust, surrender, contentment, gratitude, service, open-mindedness, and willingness. Perhaps, because my thinking inclines toward complicating matters, it was just too simple and straightforward for me to comprehend that spiritual principles don't have to be complex and mystical. I know better now. I maintain awareness that humility is not thinking less of myself, just thinking of myself less, and that self-compassion and self-forgiveness are spiritual principles that I deserve to practice.

Compassion for others means recognizing their suffering and experiencing a heart-based response to their pain. It evokes an interest in helping to ameliorate their suffering—for example, offering understanding and kindness to others when they struggle, make mistakes, or fail. Compassion is a spiritual experience with a spillover effect; compassion breeds more compassion. Recent scientific research provides evidence that the experience of compassion toward a single individual facilitates compassion toward others.[27] Empirical data also demonstrates that our sense of compassion increases measurably when we can find commonality and connection with others.[28]

Compassion radiates whenever we can connect with another through shared experience. This can take many forms, including the awareness that suffering, failure, and imperfection are universal to the experience of being. As Pema Chödrön, an American Buddhist nun and a leading teacher of Tibetan Buddhism in the West has put it, "Compassion becomes real when we recognize our shared humanity. Only when we know our own darkness well can we be present with the darkness of others."

Self-compassion consists of responding the same way toward myself when I have a difficult time, make mistakes, act out on my personality challenges, or experience something I don't like about myself. Instead of harshly judging and criticizing myself for my inadequacies, I try to be kind and understanding with myself. Because I can't ignore my pain and feel compassion for it at the same time, self-compassion requires holding my distressing thoughts, emotions, and physical sensations in mindful awareness. Perhaps most importantly, having compassion for myself means that I honor my humanness by accepting myself when I bump up against my limitations and fall short of my ideals.

The more I can open my heart to the reality that pain and inadequacy are things that everyone goes through instead of fighting against it, the more I am able to practice compassion for myself and others. As the *Tao Te Ching* states in Verse 67, "Compassionate toward yourself, you reconcile all beings in the world." This changes how I act. In applying humility, open-mindedness, empathy, and compassion in my dealings with others, I try to remember to ask myself: Is what I have in mind to say true? Is it necessary that I say it? And can I say it with kindness? If the answer to these questions isn't yes, it gives me pause to consciously consider whether what I was going to say is better left unsaid.

The head separates; the heart connects. Notice what happens when you exercise these and other spiritual principles in your interactions with other people. When we act differently toward others, they tend to act differently toward us.

Change produces myriad ripple effects; the more significant the change, the larger these ripples are. When I was presented with the chance to join Central Recovery Press, as positive and exciting as it was, and as grateful as I was for the opportunity, moving to Las Vegas did not come without serious ambivalence and costs. There was stress and anxiety about the immensity of the changes I'd be making, and great sadness regarding the significant losses of leaving Tucson—my home group, my sponsor, a number of my dearest friends on the planet, but most importantly, my younger daughter who lived with my ex-wife.

The idea of living so far away from her tore me up. The final death rattles of my active addiction followed by my stay in treatment and the divorce had left her with a sense of emotional abandonment. But at least I was still able to spend time with her regularly and be there for her literally, even if we no longer lived under the same roof. Moving out of state would put considerable geographic distance between us and add physical abandonment to an already complex and confusing mix of emotions. Although the path I needed to travel was apparent, I absolutely hated the thought of adding further to her hurt.

Toward the end of our last visit before I moved, the dam holding back a vast reservoir of emotion burst and we held each other and cried together in sadness and mourning for a long time. It came in waves, lasting for what seemed like many minutes before subsiding, only to rise and crest again, and then again.

Although we stayed in close touch and had a couple of seemingly positive in-person visits, about six months after I moved, and shortly after Jimmy became my sponsor, my daughter made it clear that she no longer wanted to have anything to do with me—no contact, period. I felt as if a UFC heavyweight champion had decked me with a kidney punch.

This was my daughter who, several years before, I had asked to teach me about the Japanese anime shows with which she was so enamored. If it was that important to her, I wanted to learn about it so I could share it with her. We spent many hours together watching her favorite anime shows. I grew to enjoy them, but what I adored was being able to connect with her in this way.

Our estrangement left a gaping hole in my heart. I called her and left voicemail messages. I sent text messages. I emailed her. And there was no response—at all. All I wanted to do was find a way to fix it now, to control it. And there was nothing I could do. I was utterly powerless. Well, I was powerless to make it better—what I did have was the capacity to further fuck it up. I was aware that the harder I tried to fix the situation, the more likely I was to make it worse. I knew full well that the worst-case scenario would be for me to react based on my emotional pain and give my personality challenges access to the driver's seat of my behavior.

Grief and sadness morphed into frustration and anger and back into grief and sadness, along with feelings of abject failure. I consulted closely with Jimmy, who had had similar adventures with his own daughter. He counseled patience and acceptance—with respect to the circumstances beyond my control and my emotional responses to them. As he put it, "We recover through our feelings. We need to embrace them, sit with them, and meditate on them, however uncomfortable or painful they may be, in order to make peace with and accept them."

I had to consciously acknowledge and accept my own pain in order to be fully present with the pain of my daughter. I continued to leave her messages at regular intervals via text, email, and voicemail, but I let go of my emotional attachment to a reply from her. Through my actions, I was committed to letting her know that I loved her and that I wasn't going anywhere, and reinforcing that I would be here for her—whenever she was ready—no matter what. I had no idea when that might be. I had no viable alternative but to give time (and my daughter) whatever time was necessary. Although there were periods when I was fearful as to how long it might be before there was any rapprochement between us or whether there would ever be one, somehow I was able to trust that the process would work out the way it needed to. I was able to mobilize enough faith to believe that it would ultimately be okay.

After nearly a year had passed, my daughter sent word through her mother that she didn't want me to attend her high school graduation in Tucson. As crushed as I was, I was more distraught that I was still a source of so much pain for her. As badly as I wanted to be there (I had never before missed a milestone event in the lives of my children), I had to respect her request. I continued to leave messages that I hoped she was okay and that I loved her. Despite the tumult in other areas of her life, she completed high school with a nearly 4.0 GPA, and several months later, started college at Northern Arizona University in Flagstaff with a full tuition scholarship.

Early in her first semester I emailed my daughter asking if it would be okay for me to come visit her at college. I had hopes, but no expectations. Three weeks later I was on my way to Flagstaff, my cheeks streaked with tears of gratitude, to see her for the first time in seventeen months. Flagstaff is a scenic three-and-a-half hour drive from Vegas that takes one southeast over the Colorado River to Kingman, AZ, and west on Interstate 40. I-40 cuts across northern Arizona, passing the tiny rural communities of Seligman, Ash Fork, and Williams (the self-proclaimed "Gateway to the Grand Canyon"), as it bisects expansive meadows and gradually rises in elevation through ecosystems that transition from Juniper trees and Pinyon pines at 4,000–5,000 feet to evergreen forests at 6,000–7,000 feet. Flagstaff is a quintessential college town with a population of approximately 60,000 and a vibrant downtown nestled among the evergreens at 6,900 feet above sea level.

I've become intimately familiar with all 249 miles of that drive. It didn't happen all at once, but I have been able to rebuild my relationship with my younger daughter. In the winter of 2011, her mother moved from Tucson to the Midwest for a sensational new job, leaving me by far her most local parent. Being able to be here for her is a beautiful thing. Having both of my now adult daughters in my life is a blessing beyond description.

In the midst of stressful and emotionally charged circumstances, confounding thoughts and discombobulating emotions can swirl around us at hurricane speed. It can be easy to get swept away by the intensity of such gale force winds. And yet, it doesn't have to happen. By practicing the skills and spiritual principles of recovery, I am able to find refuge and spend more time in the eye of such emotional hurricanes, where there is relative quiet and calm.

I try to act the way I want to be, and gradually I become the way I act. Learning life one day at a time challenges the internal perfectionist's impossible demands. Guilt-tripping, shame-inducing, crazy-making voices whose siren seductions began so long ago in galaxies so far away still occasionally call me collect. With each step I take along this path, these noises with their spirit-suffocating lies grow less insistent and less influential, as self-recrimination slowly subsides. Increasingly, I am okay being perfectly imperfect.

The more that I can remain in conscious contact with spiritual principles, the more mindful and present-centered I am. It turns out that the only way to fill internal emptiness is from the inside out. My experience, in combination with the experience, strength, and hope shared by many others, has led me to the clear realization that there are no external solutions to internal challenges. Recovery really is an "inside" job. The mere fact of my continuing recovery from addiction and chronic pain represents a huge spiritual awakening: never in my wildest pre-treatment imaginings did I believe it would be possible for me to live without the use of drugs, period. Never mind doing so in the presence of chronic pain.

The unfolding of spiritual awakenings to me is similar to the process of dying cloth. Let's say that I want to change the color of a piece of white cloth to a dark royal blue. The cloth is white (no shit) and the container of dye is a deep, rich blue. If I am new to this process, I might expect that as soon as the cloth hits the dye it will turn the desired color. Yet, the first time the cloth is put into the dye it may just barely change color, to a very faint blue. It is only by continuing to dip the cloth into the dye over and over again that the color changes noticeably. Each time the cloth comes in contact with the dye, the color becomes a little deeper and richer.

While the difference in color from the very beginning of the process is clear and dramatic, the difference from one repetition of dipping to the next may be so slight that it's difficult to notice. And so it has been with most of the spiritual awakenings I have experienced. I have to keep putting my ass (so to speak) into the dye that is my program of recovery in order to get the results I am seeking—deepened spirituality and an enriched quality of life.

chapter nineteen

[THERE IS NO GRADUATION]

"Behold this day . . . it is yours to make."
BLACK ELK, OGLALA SIOUX LAKOTA MEDICINE MAN

I noted earlier that as hard as it is to stop using and become abstinent, it is a much more formidable challenge to stay stopped and remain abstinent by learning and practicing how to live without the use of mind- and mood-altering substances. Recovery from addiction—with or without chronic pain as a co-occurring disorder—is the process of sustaining abstinence *and* learning and practicing the awareness and skills necessary to live a whole, healthy, and healed life. These two elements reinforce one another: sustained abstinence creates the opportunities to learn and practice the skills that facilitate growth and healing, which is not possible during the unremitting entropy of active addiction. Conversely, learning and practicing the skills that facilitate growth and healing is instrumental to sustaining abstinence.

Without abstinence, recovery is not possible. However, and as I have described throughout this book, recovery is much more than simply remaining abstinent from the specific manifestations of one's addiction. Abstinence is the avoidance of the objects of one's addiction, whether they be drugs and/or activities. Beyond abstinence, recovery is

- participating in life activities that are healthy, meaningful, and fulfilling based on my needs and interests;

- changing my attitudes and my actions, as well as my relationship to my thoughts and emotions, especially those that are uncomfortable and painful;

- discovering parts of myself of which I had been unaware, and rediscovering those parts of myself that were buried in the rubble of active addiction;

- learning and practicing new patterns of living, finding new meaning in life, and moving toward physical, mental, emotional, and spiritual balance.

Every once in a while, well-meaning people outside the world of recovery have asked me when I will "graduate" or how long will it be before I'm "recovered" or "cured" and no longer "have to go to those meetings." I'm grateful that there is no graduation from recovery. It is a lifelong, one day at a time process that can only happen in the unfurling of each moment. Recovery provides by far my best chance to live a whole, healthy, and healed life. Why wouldn't I want to continue to walk this path? I can think of no good enough reasons.

Twelve-step addiction recovery programs are sometimes criticized for perceived low rates of success—as defined by the percentage of people who start attending meetings compared with those who remain abstinent and in recovery over time. Addiction is a chronic, progressive, and potentially fatal illness, similar to other chronic life-threatening diseases such as Type 2 diabetes, asthma, and hypertension. Just like these other diseases, there is no cure; compliance with treatment protocols is often inconsistent, and relapse is all too common.

The reality is that the vast majority of people basically pass by or pass through these programs, never making a serious commitment to recovery. A drive-by approach to recovery won't get it done. Recovery that's built to last requires perseverance. It's a lot of work, and in order to be successful, a person really has to want it. Practicing addicts typically devote multiple hours each day to maintaining their active addiction—planning and pursuing the ways and means to use, using, and recovering from the acute effects of using. Most give little thought to the significant amount of time and energy it takes to support their addiction—they simply do what they have to do. Yet, many of these same individuals become extremely concerned about the amount of time and energy maintaining recovery requires, and are ultimately unwilling to make that investment.

In my experience—both professional and personal—anyone willing to allocate just 25–50 percent of the time, attention, and energy to recovery that he or she previously spent chasing his or her active addiction will have excellent opportunities to be successful. Among those who commit themselves to recovery and remain committed, by putting their actions where their mouths are, the rate of success I have observed is impressive (though I couldn't responsibly put a percentage on it) and presents a fertile topic for scientific study.

My program of recovery works, but only *if* I work it. I have access to a remarkable structure for growth and healing and a system of support that is second to none, but the bottom line is that no one else can do for me what I am unwilling to do for myself. After all, as my friend Connie is fond of saying, it's a fucking *self-help* program!

For people in recovery, the potential for relapse is a reality, but relapse is not a requirement. There are no small number of people who make the decision to change their lives and seek recovery, and never use again.

To this point, I am one of them, though I know full well that no one is immune to the possibility of relapse.

In the field of addiction treatment, the topic of relapse prevention receives considerable attention at all levels of care. However, the rubric of relapse prevention may not be the most therapeutic way to frame the life-affirming value of moving further away from active addiction and toward recovery. We instinctively hear "positive" messages as to what to do more readily than "negative" messages admonishing us what not to do. I believe it's more helpful to emphasize what to embrace as opposed to what to avoid.

For me, the key to relapse prevention is the maintenance of my recovery. Such maintenance is not an every-once-in-a-while episode; it is an ongoing, daily process. Steps Ten, Eleven, and Twelve are known as the "maintenance steps." Recovery maintenance is a lot like tending a garden. If I want healthy results, it requires consistent attention and concerted effort—tilling the soil, careful planting, checking for and pulling weeds, and regular watering—in short, continuing attention, care, and feeding. I need to make adjustments in the care I provide in response to changing conditions, such as seasonal fluctuations and episodic shifts in rainfall, temperature, etc. If we want something/anything to last, we need to take good care of it. This process is artfully detailed (albeit using a different metaphor) in that classic piece of 1970's literature, *Zen and the Art of Motorcycle Maintenance.*

Contrary to popular misconception, relapse doesn't begin with a return to using; using is the culmination of the relapse process, a process that usually starts long before the resumption of the actual use of substances or other manifestations of addiction. The seeds for a return to using are sown during a gradual return to the same kinds of thinking, attitudes, ways of dealing (or not dealing) with feelings, and behaviors that pervaded active addiction. The onset of this relapse process frequently begins with complacency.

Complacency refers to a sense of self-satisfaction combined with a lack of awareness of potential or actual dangers. When things appear to be going smoothly, whether in life in general, or in specific life areas (such as recovery), it can be easy to begin to take success for granted and become complacent. There is an almost natural tendency to become complacent and coast in one's recovery when all is well and seemingly going smoothly. The indicators of complacency can be shrouded by the mists of our defense mechanisms, notably a re-emergence of denial, minimization, and rationalization. However, the warning signs are apparent if we know what to look for. They include, but are not limited to:

- Believing that I have "completed" my recovery or that I am "recovered."

- Believing that I "have this recovery thing down," and know everything I need to know.

- Believing that it's been long enough that I no longer have a problem with addiction or that the amount of time I have in recovery or what I know somehow inoculates me from relapse.

- Disengaging from actively practicing the awareness and actions of recovery by significantly reducing or discontinuing going to meetings, aftercare/therapy, meditation, prayer, exercising mindfulness, applying spiritual principles, keeping in contact with one's support group, reading recovery literature, doing twelve-step work, or continuing to work with a sponsor.

- Engaging in thoughts, attitudes, and/or behaviors that were part of one's patterns in active addiction, including returning, perhaps slowly and gradually, to being involved with "people, places, and things" associated with one's using.

I've heard the relapse stories of dozens of people with long-term recovery—five, ten, fifteen, in some cases, even twenty or more years. They all seem to begin the same way and follow a consistent trajectory.

Their connection to their recovery program decreased progressively until it ceased to exist. They gradually discontinued doing the things that enabled and sustained their recovery, shedding them piece by piece—attending twelve-step meetings, contacting their sponsor, applying the steps in their daily lives, and being of service to their community.

One of the very few constants in life is change. Because change is generally perceived as arduous, it becomes anxiety-provoking and there is a natural human tendency to resist it. Recovery is a process of ongoing change that necessitates going beyond the boundaries of the containers of comfort and attachment that we have constructed for ourselves. After a year-long process, in December of 2011, the Substance Abuse and Mental Health Services Administration (SAMHSA) of the US Department of Health and Human Services, released their working definition of recovery from addiction and/or mental illness: "A process of change through which individuals improve their health and wellness, live a self-directed life, and strive to reach their full potential."

My recovery process has given me the opportunity and ability to make amends by acknowledging and taking responsibility for the harm I've caused others. However, the most meaningful amends I can make is an ongoing living amends by consciously and consistently practicing the spiritual principles that, bit-by-bit, bring me closer to the person I was intended to be, the person I want to be.

As Benjamin Franklin put it, "When you're finished changing, you're finished." The acceptance of things as they really are, as opposed to how I want them to be, or think they "should" be, is a forever process. The solution lies in continuing to utilize and build upon the resources and experiences that make it possible for me to learn and grow and heal.

Step Twelve has three elements. In addition to the spiritual awakening detailed in the last chapter, it speaks to helping transmit the message of recovery to other addicts, and practicing the principles of the Twelve Steps in all areas of our lives. Carrying the message of recovery to others involves being of service within the program. This can take many different forms—from the very simple and concrete to the sophisticated, and includes tasks that cover the entire spectrum of experience in recovery, from those who are brand new to people who have been in recovery for decades.

When one of my friends shares his experience, strength, and hope with other addicts, he often asks for a show of hands from those in the audience with at least a year in recovery. He then asks for a show of hands from everyone involved in twelve-step service work. There is generally (at minimum) a 90–95 percent overlap between these two groups. Is this merely coincidence? I think not. It is intriguing grist for empirical research, but ample anecdotal evidence suggests there is a significant correlation between the people who perform service work and those who stay in recovery.

The paradox of Step Twelve is that through the act of giving, we receive. I have been of service in my twelve-step fellowship, in a variety of roles, since four months into my recovery. Being of service is both a responsibility and a privilege. My service commitments are at night after work or on the weekends, and it is not unusual after a full day of work or when I'm chilling on the weekend, to not "feel like going." But I go, and I invariably feel better afterward. It is a giving of spirit that takes me out of myself and diffuses self-centeredness. Service simultaneously allows me to pay back what I've been given and pay it forward to others.

Occasionally I have heard people share in twelve-step meetings that "My worst day clean is better than my best day using." Say what? My reaction to that is immediate and two-fold: disbelief or sympathy. Either they are full of shit and just trying to say the "right" thing, or I feel sorry for them because they obviously didn't have access to the same quality of dope that I used. I had plenty of days using that were light years better than my "worst day clean." I had many ecstatic drug-fueled experiences. I had a massive amount of fun. Then I passed a tipping point where it became a little less fun with each time I used, as the dynamics of diminishing returns took firm hold. Eventually it wasn't fun at all; just fucked up, and

I had to find a new way to live. There are times when life on its own terms still kicks my ass. Life in recovery doesn't necessarily get easier, but it does get better.

Success is no accident. Although, obviously there are exceptions, generally people do not experience serious problems in living, including addiction, by accident or coincidence. Our choices and actions—both conscious and unconscious—contribute to the vast majority of the problems we experience, including those related to active addiction. In the same way, success also happens as a result of the choices people make and the actions they take.

We are defined less by our abilities than by the choices we make and the actions we take in support of those choices. Learning how to identify the ingredients that help us successfully maintain recovery is an important skill. Because when we can identify the specific ingredients of success in any area of our lives, we can then translate that awareness into action, and take the steps to recreate or continue that success.

For many years, I've worn a pendant crafted by a Hopi silver and goldsmith. I was drawn to its beauty and symbolism, but its meaning has only become more resonant since I've been in recovery. "The Man in the Maze," is an ancient symbol of the Tohono O'odham Nation of southern Arizona and northern Sonora, Mexico. Said to represent a person's journey through life, this symbol is used in silversmithing and basket weaving in several Native American cultures of the American Southwest. The intricate maze signifies the difficult journey toward finding deeper meaning in life. Sharp twists and turns denote decision points, struggles, lessons learned, and choices made along the way.

Big successes rarely occur all at once. They are almost always built on a foundation of small successes. There are plenty of stories of bands who play together for a decade, develop their style and work their asses off, drive their own beat-up vehicles from one small, lousy-paying gig to another to play in front of audiences that begin as tiny but grow over time, who suddenly become "overnight successes." Successful long-term recovery is built similarly—one day at a time. As the Tao Te Ching, states in Verse 63, "accomplish the great task by a series of small acts."

At its core, recovery is about reclaiming one's humanity and reconnecting with one's true self. For D. W. Winnicott, the "false self" that evolves unconsciously in earliest childhood to accommodate the demands of one's family environment, especially primary caregivers, is contrasted with the "true self." The true self is the instinctive essence of our persona; the innate capacity to know and operationalize our natural individual needs for self-expression and self-fulfillment. The true self is the self at its most genuine, opening the door to true intimacy with others, as well as congruence between who I am on the inside and how I act on the outside, and across different areas of my life, from one setting to another.

The concept of the true self fits with what Carl Rogers described as the built-in motivation present in every organism to develop its potential to the fullest extent possible—an "actualizing tendency." This actualizing tendency grows people's capacity to lead lives that are authentic and ingenuous. I believe that in every circumstance, people do the best they can, based on their current capacity. Through recovery our capacity expands; it becomes greater, enhancing our conscious access to resources, and making more options and possibilities available to us. Recovery unchains our actualizing tendency, unearthing the rediscovery of true self.

Gabor Maté, MD, is a physician who specializes in addiction treatment and works with the most down-and-out hardcore drug addicts in Vancouver, British Columbia. He describes addiction as the antithesis of peace, a disconnection from the self that creates great internal unrest. For Dr. Maté, healing means to become whole and recovery is about finding oneself. He notes the commonality between the Hebrew words for wholeness—*shalem* and peace—*shalom*, to conclude that when we find ourselves and become whole, we can find peace.

Recovery from addiction and chronic pain is a never-ending undertaking that involves coming to terms with myself exactly as I am, and accepting life on its own terms with its full range of pain and pleasure, while expanding my capacity to act consciously rather than react habitually and reflexively. It is about making conscious decisions consistent with what I value most and taking action to spend my available energy and precious time in ways that accurately reflect my priorities. Recovery is a path of wisdom guided by mindfully acknowledging and living fully in this moment, accepting myself with all of my imperfections. This is incredibly challenging, and I know most people struggle mightily in their attempts at it. Yet people do it everyday.

Early in my clinical training, when I was learning how to distinguish between my ass and third base as far as psychotherapy, I was surprised to hear even extremely experienced and skilled therapists (some of whom seemed to have real mastery of the craft) state straightforwardly that there were times when they had no clear idea "what was happening in the room." In other words, in those moments, they were confused and unsure about what was going on in their therapy with a given client. However, if they hung in there, exercising patience while continuing to be present-centered and emotionally available, the issues would clarify and they would find their way back to being in sync with the therapeutic process.

The same dynamic operates in the process of recovery—sometimes things are unclear and confused and confusing. Rather than getting twisted up because I'm struggling and may not know what the hell is going on, if I hang in there and remain mindfully accepting, open to possibility, and patient—the mud will settle and the water will become clear again.

Assembling the pieces that sustain recovery and nurture a life of meaning, contentment, and value is a continuous process. It requires identifying and gathering the necessary pieces, seeing how they fit together, and often reconfiguring them—replacing some pieces with others and rearranging them to create the most functional and healthy fit. This fit is individualized; what fits beautifully for me may not be a great fit for you, and vice-versa. Sometimes we put the pieces together and they seem to work well for a time. After being in place for a while they may not work so well, and we modify them or seek out new pieces or a different configuration that fits and works better for us.

When I was Clinical Director of the Chemical Dependency Unit at Good Samaritan Hospital in Suffern, New York, for those five years in the mid-1990s, I worked closely with the program's medical director. He was a psychiatrist who was in recovery for quite a few years through the "founding" twelve-step fellowship. He was brilliant, quick to anger, and so compassionate with our patients that it sometimes created conflict with more law-and-order-oriented staff. In spite of every-once-in-a-while outbursts of upset, he was a quiet and gentle man who rarely mentioned his own recovery.

At one of the many professional conferences on addiction that I attended, he gave a talk that focused on his personal recovery experience. During a powerful and moving presentation, he described being grateful that he was an alcoholic. He went on to say that, in contrast to most people who operate more or less on automatic pilot and effectively sleepwalk through life, embarking on a process of recovery had given him the awareness to live life much more intentionally. As a result, he took little for granted and appreciated much. Although his reasoning made sense, it was difficult for me to wrap my mind (never mind my heart) around the idea of having such profound gratitude for being an addict . . . until I found my way to my own recovery.

Life takes its toll on all of us, and everyone, whether or not they struggle with addiction, chronic pain, or any other serious condition, sustains a certain degree of damage along the way. The rooms of recovery are full of damaged people—some of whom have been abused and traumatized in horrific ways. Recovery provides a pathway to heal from that damage, to become stronger, just as broken bones can become stronger after they heal than they were prior to injury. It is a warrior's path that requires strength and courage to traverse. Every step along the way is a step toward grace.

Everything is interconnected, and I can connect virtually anything to my process of recovery. Sometimes these linkages are direct and unmistakable; sometimes they are mitigated by degrees of separation that require more effort to uncover. Every experience has something to teach me. Lessons abound and opportunities for growth and healing come in many different shapes and sizes. Whenever my mind and heart are open enough, I find those lessons. The assembly of these physical, mental, emotional, and spiritual parts creates a whole infinitely greater than their sum, releasing the revelation of a true self that was well hidden, but always there—waiting to greet me.

[ENDNOTES]

[1] Substance Abuse and Mental Health Services Administration, *Results from the 2010 National Survey on Drug Use and Health: Volume 1: Summary of National Findings* (Rockville, MD: Substance Abuse and Mental Health Services Administration, Office of Applied Studies, 2011), accessed December 11, 2012, http://oas.samhsa.gov/ NSDUH/2k10NSDUH/2k10Results.htm#2.16.

[2] Lisa Girion, Scott Glover, and Doug Smith, "Drug Deaths Now Outnumber Traffic Fatalities in U.S., Data Show," *Los Angeles Times*, September 17, 2011, http://articles.latimes.com/2011/sep/17/local/ la-me-drugs-epidemic-20110918.

[3] Pain–76.2 million people, National Centers for Health Statistics: Diabetes–20.8 million people (diagnosed and estimated undiagnosed), American Diabetes Association; Coronary Heart Disease (including heart attack and chest pain) and Stroke–18.7 million people, American Heart Association; Cancer–1.4 million people, American Cancer Society.

[4] National Center for Health Statistics, *Health, United States, 2006:* "With Chart Book on Trends in the Health of Americans with Special Feature on Pain" (CDC National Center for Health Statistics Press, 2006).

[5] National Institutes of Health, NIH Guide: "New Directions in Pain Research I," September 4, 1998, http://grants.nih.gov/grants/guide/pa-files/PA-98-102.html.

[6] Centers for Disease Control and Prevention, "Policy Impact: Prescription Painkiller Overdoses," November 2011, http://www.cdc.gov/ homeandrecreationalsafety/rxbrief/.

[7] Substance Abuse and Mental Health Services Administration, *Results from the 2010 National Survey on Drug Use and Health: Volume 1: Summary of National Findings* (Rockville, MD: Substance Abuse and Mental Health Services Administration, Office of Applied Studies, 2011), http://oas.samhsa.gov/NSDUH/2k10NSDUH/2k10Results.htm#2.16, accessed December 11, 2012.

[8] Substance Abuse and Mental Health Services Administration, Drug Abuse Warning Network: "Selected Tables of National Estimates of Drug-Related Emergency Department Visits" (Rockville, MD: Center for Behavioral Health Statistics and Quality, SAMHSA, 2010).

[9] *Narcotics Anonymous*, 6th ed. (Chatsworth, CA: Narcotics Anonymous World Services, Inc.; 2008), 65.

[10] N. D. Volkow et al, "Loss of Dopamine Transporters in Methamphetamine Abusers Recovers with Protracted Abstinence," *Journal of Neuroscience* 21, no. 23 (2001): 9414–9418.

[11] B. Ivanovski and G. S. Malhi, "The Psychological and Neurophysiological Concomitants of Mindfulness Forms of Meditation," *Acta Neurpsychiatrica* 19, no. 76 (2007): 76–91.

[12] S. Bowen et al, "The Role of Thought Suppression in the Relationship Between Mindfulness Meditation and Alcohol Use," *Addictive Behaviors* 32 (2007): 2324–28.

[13] Gaëlle Desbordes et al, "Effects of Mindful-Attention and Compassion Meditation Training on Amygdala Response to Emotional Stimuli in an Ordinary, Non-Meditative State," *Frontiers in Human Neuroscience* 6 (2012): 292.

[14] M. J. Cooper et al, "Transcendental Meditation in the Management of Hypercholesterolemia," *Journal of Human Stress* 5 (1979): 24–27; M. J. Cooper and M. M. Aygen, "Effect of Transcendental Meditation on Serum Cholesterol and Blood Pressure," *Harefuah, Journal of the Israel Medical Association* 95 (1978): 1–2.

[15] Maura Paul-Labrador et al, "Effects of a Randomized Controlled Trial of Transcendental Meditation on Components of the Metabolic Syndrome in Subjects With Coronary Heart Disease," *Archives of Internal Medicine* 166 (2006): 1218–24.

[16] J. W. Anderson et al, "Blood Pressure Response to Transcendental Meditation: A Meta-Analysis," *American Journal of Hypertension* 21 (2008): 310–16.

[17] R. H. Schneider et al, "Long-Term Effects of Stress Reduction on Mortality in Persons > or = 55 Years of Age With Systemic Hypertension," *American Journal of Cardiology* 95 (2005): 1060–64.

[18] A. Newberg and J. Iverson, "The Neural Basis of the Complex Mental Task of Meditation: Neurotransmitter and Neurochemical Consideration," *Medical Hypotheses* 61, no. 2 (August 2003): 282–91.

[19] G. Pagoni and M. Cekic, "Age Effects on Gray Matter Volume and Attentional Performance in Zen Meditation," *Neurobiology of Aging* 28, no. 10 (2007): 1623–27.

[20] Eileen Luders et al, "Enhanced Brain Connectivity in Long-Term Meditation Practitioners," *Neuroimage* 57, no. 4 (August 2011): 1308–16.

[21] F. Zeidan et al, "Brain Mechanisms Supporting the Modulation of Pain by Mindfulness Meditation," *Journal of Neuroscience* 31, no. 14 (April 2011): 5540–48.

[22] John Muir, *Our National Parks* (Boston and New York: Houghton, Mifflin, and Company, 1901), 56.

[23] John Muir, *My First Summer in the Sierra* (Boston and New York: Houghton, Mifflin, and Company, 1911), 19.

[24] S. Carroll, "Spirituality and Purpose in Life in Alcoholism Recovery," *Journal of Studies on Alcohol and Drugs* 54 (May 1993): 297–301.

[25] James E. Corrington, "Spirituality and Recovery: Relationships Between Levels of Spirituality, Contentment and Stress During Recovery from Alcoholism in AA," *Alcohol Treatment Quarterly* 6, no. 3–4 (1989): 151–65.

[26] J. M. White, R. S. Wampler, and J. L. Fischer, "Indicators of Spiritual Development in Recovery from Alcohol and Other Drug Problems," *Alcohol Treatment Quarterly* 19 (2001): 19–35.

[27] Paul Condon and David DeSteno, "Compassion For One Reduces Punishment For Another," *Journal of Experimental Social Psychology* 47, no. 3 (2011): 698–701.

[28] Piercarlo Valdesolo and David DeSteno, "Synchrony and the Social Tuning of Compassion," *Emotion* 11, no. 2 (2011): 262–66.

[REFERENCES]

Addiction Technology Transfer Center (ATTC) website:
http://www.attcnetwork.org/explore/priorityareas/science/

American Psychiatric Association. *Diagnostic and Statistical Manual of Mental Disorders:* 4th ed. Washington, DC: American Psychiatric Association, 1994.

Ash, Mel. *The Zen of Recovery.* New York: Jeremy P. Tarcher/ Putnam, 1993.

Black, Claudia. *It Will Never Happen to Me: Growing Up With Addiction As Youngsters, Adolescents, Adults.* 2nd ed. Center City, MN: Hazelden, 2002.

Black, Claudia. *Repeat After Me.* 2nd rev. ed. Denver: Medical Administration Co, 1995.

Chödrön, Pema. *The Places that Scare You: A Guide to Fearlessness in Difficult Times.* Boston: Shambhala Publications, 2001.

Dass, Ram. *Remember, Be Here Now.* San Cristobal, NM: Lama Foundation, 1971.

Ellis, Albert. *Anger: How to Live With and Without It.* Rev. ed. New York: Citadel Press Books, 2003.

Epstein, Mark. *Open to Desire: The Truth about What the Buddha Taught.* New York: Penguin Group (USA) Inc., 2006.

Epstein, Mark. *Thoughts Without A Thinker: Psychotherapy from a Buddhist Perspective.* New York: Basic Books, 2004.

Erikson, E. H. *Childhood and Society*. New York: W. W. Norton, 1950.

Erikson, E. H. *Identity: Youth and Crisis*. New York: W. W. Norton, 1968.

Erickson, Milton H. *The Collected Works of Milton H. Erickson. Vol. 10, Hypnotic Realities: The Induction of Clinical Hypnosis and Forms of Indirect Suggestion*. Edited by L. Rossi, Roxanna Erickson-Klein, and Kathryn Lane Rossi. Phoenix, AZ: The Milton H. Erickson Foundation Press, 2010.

Frankl, Viktor. *Man's Search for Meaning*. Boston: Beacon Press, 2006. (Dr. Frankl completed the book in 1946, and it eventually reached an enormous general readership around the world. At the time of his death in 1997 at the age of 92, it had been reprinted 73 times, and translated into 24 languages.)

Gatchel, R. J. and K. H. Rollings. "Evidence-Informed Management of Chronic Low Back Pain with Cognitive Behavioral Therapy." *The Spine Journal* 8, no. 1 (2008): 40–4.

Havens, Ronald. *The Wisdom of Milton H. Erickson: The Complete Volume.* Carmarthen, Wales: Crown House Publishing, 2005.

Hayes, S. C., K. Strosahl, and K. G. Wilson. *Acceptance and Commitment Therapy: The Process and Practice of Mindful Change*. 2nd ed. New York: Guilford Press, 2011.

Kabat-Zinn, Jon. *Full Catastrophe Living: Using the Wisdom of Your Body and Mind to Face Stress, Pain, and Illness.* New York: Delacorte Press, 1990.

O'Hanlon, Bill. *Taproots: Underlying Principles of Milton Erickson's Therapy and Hypnosis*. New York: W. W. Norton & Company, 1981.

Lao Tzu. *Tao Te Ching*. Translated by Stephen Mitchell. New York: Harper and Row, 1988.

Linehan, Marsha M. *Skills Training Manual for Treating Borderline Personality Disorder.* New York: Guilford Press, 1993.

Maté, Gabor. *Close Encounters with Addiction.* Las Vegas: Central Recovery Press, 2011. E-book.

Narcotics Anonymous. *It Works How and Why: The Twelve Steps and Twelve Traditions of Narcotics Anonymous*. Chatsworth, CA: Narcotics Anonymous World Services, Inc., 1993.

Narcotics Anonymous. *Narcotics Anonymous*. 6th ed. Chatsworth, CA: Narcotics Anonymous World Services, Inc., 2008.

National Institute on Drug Abuse. *Drugs, Brains, and Behavior: The Science of Addiction*. National Institute on Drug Abuse, 2007. Revised 2010. http://drugabuse.gov/scienceofaddiction/sciofaddiction.pdf.

National Institute on Drug Abuse. "NIDA-Supported Researchers Use Brain Imaging to Deepen Understanding of Addiction." *NIDA Notes Special Report: Brain Imaging Research* 11, no. 5 (November/December 1996).

Pohl, Mel. *A Day without Pain*. Rev. ed. Las Vegas: Central Recovery Press, 2011.

Pohl, Mel, Frank J. Szabo, Daniel Shiode, and Robert Hunter. *Pain Recovery: How to Find Balance and Reduce Suffering from Chronic Pain*. Las Vegas: Central Recovery Press, 2009.

Rogers, Carl. *Client-Centered Therapy: Its Current Practice, Implications and Theory*. London: Constable, 1951.

Schenck, Nancy. *Tails of Recovery: Addicts and the Pets That Love Them*. Las Vegas: Central Recovery Press, 2009.

Schneider, Jennifer P. "Addiction and Chronic Pain." The National Pain Foundation. January 2009. http://www.nationalpainfoundation.org/articles/134/addiction-and-chronic-pain.

Substance Abuse and Mental Health Services Administration, Office of Applied Studies. *Results from the 2009 National Survey on Drug Use and Health: National Findings*. 2010.

The Editors of Central Recovery Press. *Recovery A to Z: A Handbook of Twelve-Step Key Terms and Phrases*. 2nd ed. Las Vegas: Central Recovery Press, 2011.

Turner, Kielty. "Mindfulness: The Present Moment in Clinical Social Work." *Journal of Clinical Social Work* 37 (2009): 95–103.

Watts, Alan W. *Psychotherapy East and West.* New York: Random House, 1975.

Wegscheider-Cruse, Sharon. *Another Chance: Hope and Health for the Alcoholic Family.* Deerfield Beach, FL: Health Communications, Inc., 1989.

Winnicott, D. W. *The Child, the Family, and the Outside World.* Middlesex, England: Pelican Books, 1973.

Winnicott, D. W. "Ego Distortion in Terms of True and False Self." In *The Maturational Processes and the Facilitating Environment: Studies in the Theory of Emotional Development*, 140–152. London: Hogarth Press, 1965.

Winnicott, D. W. *Playing and Reality.* London: Tavistock, 1971.